Neuro-Ophthalmology

Editor

ANDREW G. LEE

NEUROLOGIC CLINICS

www.neurologic.theclinics.com

Consulting Editor

RANDOLPH W. EVANS

February 2017 • Volume 35 • Number 1

ELSEVIER

1600 John F. Kennedy Boulevard • Suite 1800 • Philadelphia, Pennsylvania, 19103-2899

http://www.theclinics.com

NEUROLOGIC CLINICS Volume 35, Number 1
February 2017 ISSN 0733-8619, ISBN-13: 978-0-323-49665-0

Editor: Stacy Eastman
Developmental editor: Donald Mumford

Neurologic Clinics (ISSN 0733-8619) is published quarterly by Elsevier Inc., 360 Park Avenue South, New York, NY 10010–1710. Months of issue are February, May, August, and November. Periodicals postage paid at New York, NY, and additional mailing offices. Subscription prices are $306.00 per year for US individuals, $607.00 per year for US institutions, $100.00 per year for US students, $383.00 per year for Canadian individuals, $736.00 per year for Canadian institutions, $423.00 per year for international individuals, $736.00 per year for international institutions, and $210.00 for Canadian and foreign students/residents. To receive student/resident rate, orders must be accompanied by name of affiliated institution, date of term, and the *signature* of program/residency coordinator on institution letterhead. Orders will be billed at individual rate until proof of status is received. Foreign air speed delivery is included in all *Clinics* subscription prices. All prices are subject to change without notice. **POSTMASTER:** Send address changes to *Neurologic Clinics*, Elsevier Health Sciences Division, Subscription Customer Service, 3251 Riverport Lane, Maryland Heights, MO 63043. **Customer Service: Telephone: 1-800-654-2452 (U.S. and Canada); 314-447-8871 (outside U.S. and Canada). Fax: 314-447-8029. E-mail: journalscustomerservice-usa@elsevier.com (for print support); journalsonlinesupport-usa@elsevier.com (for online support).**

Reprints. For copies of 100 or more of articles in this publication, please contact the Commercial Reprints Department, Elsevier Inc., 360 Park Avenue South, New York, New York, 10010-1710; Tel.: +1-212-633-3874; Fax: +1-212-633-3820, and E-mail: reprints@elsevier.com.

Neurologic Clinics is also published in Spanish by Nueva Editorial Interamericana S.A., Mexico City, Mexico.

Neurologic Clinics is covered in *Current Contents/Clinical Medicine, MEDLINE/PubMed (Index Medicus), EMBASE/Excerpta Medica, and PsycINFO, and ISI/BIOMED.*

Contributors

CONSULTING EDITOR

RANDOLPH W. EVANS, MD
Clinical Professor, Department of Neurology, Baylor College of Medicine, Houston, Texas

EDITOR

ANDREW G. LEE, MD
Blanton Eye Institute of Houston Methodist Hospital, Houston, Texas; Departments of Ophthalmology, Neurology, and Neurosurgery, Weill Cornell Medical College, New York, New York; Department of Ophthalmology, University of Texas Medical Branch, Galveston, Texas; Department of Ophthalmology, University of Texas MD Anderson Cancer Center, Houston, Texas; Department of Ophthalmology, Baylor College of Medicine, Houston, Texas; Department of Ophthalmology, The University of Iowa Hospitals and Clinics, Iowa City, Iowa

AUTHORS

JOHANNA D. BEEBE, MD
Department of Ophthalmology and Visual Sciences, University of Iowa Hospitals and Clinics, Iowa City, Iowa

VALÉRIE BIOUSSE, MD
Professor of Ophthalmology and Neurology; Cyrus H. Stoner Professor of Ophthalmology; Emory University School of Medicine, Atlanta, Georgia

JESSICA R. CHANG, MD
Ophthalmology, Wilmer Eye Institute/Johns Hopkins University School of Medicine, Baltimore, Maryland

FIONA COSTELLO, MD, FRCP
Associate Professor, Departments of Clinical Neurosciences and Surgery, University of Calgary, Calgary, Alberta, Canada

MICHAEL DATTILO, MD, PhD
Department of Ophthalmology, Emory University School of Medicine; Neuro-Ophthalmology, Emory Eye Center, Atlanta, Georgia

MARC J. DINKIN, MD
Assistant Professor of Ophthalmology, Departments of Ophthalmology, Neurology and Neurosurgery, New York Presbyterian Hospital, Weill Cornell Medical College, New York, New York

JEANNE FEUERSTEIN, MD
Resident in Neurology, University of Colorado School of Medicine, Aurora, Colorado

ROD FOROOZAN, MD
Baylor College of Medicine, Houston, Texas

ALEXANDER FROLOV, MD
Resident in Neurology, University of Colorado School of Medicine, Aurora, Colorado

ANNA M. GRUENER, BMBS, MSc, FRCOphth
Ophthalmology, Wilmer Eye Institute/Johns Hopkins University School of Medicine, Baltimore, Maryland

RANDY H. KARDON, MD, PhD
Tenured Professor and Pomeranz Family Chair in Ophthalmology, Director of Neuro-Ophthalmology and Iowa City VA Center for the Prevention and Treatment of Visual Loss, Department of Ophthalmology and Visual Sciences, University of Iowa Hospitals and Clinics; Iowa City VA Medical Center, Iowa City, Iowa

ANDREW G. LEE, MD
Blanton Eye Institute of Houston Methodist Hospital, Houston, Texas; Departments of Ophthalmology, Neurology, and Neurosurgery, Weill Cornell Medical College, New York, New York; Department of Ophthalmology, University of Texas Medical Branch, Galveston, Texas; Department of Ophthalmology, University of Texas MD Anderson Cancer Center, Houston, Texas; Department of Ophthalmology, Baylor College of Medicine, Houston, Texas; Department of Ophthalmology, The University of Iowa Hospitals and Clinics, Iowa City, Iowa

TIMOTHY J. McCULLEY, MD
Vice Chair for Clinical Strategic Planning; Director, Neuro-Ophthalmology; Director, Oculoplastic Surgery at Bayview; Director, American Society Ophthalmic Plastic and Reconstructive Surgery (ASOPRS) Fellowship, Ophthalmology, Wilmer Eye Institute/ Johns Hopkins University School of Medicine, Baltimore, Maryland

NANCY J. NEWMAN, MD
Professor of Ophthalmology, Neurology and Neurosurgery; LeoDelle Jolley Professor of Ophthalmology; Emory University School of Medicine, Atlanta Georgia

ATHOS PATSALIDES, MD, MPH
Associate Professor, Division of Interventional Neuroradiology, Department of Neurological Surgery, New York Presbyterian Hospital, Weill Cornell Medical College, New York

HOWARD D. POMERANZ, MD, PhD
Associate Professor, Department of Ophthalmology, Northwell Health, Great Neck, New York

GLENN H. ROBERSON, MD
Department of Radiology, University of Alabama at Birmingham, Birmingham, Alabama

STACY V. SMITH, MD
Department of Ophthalmology, Blanton Eye Institute, Houston Methodist Hospital, Houston, Texas

PREM S. SUBRAMANIAN, MD, PhD
Professor of Ophthalmology, Neurology, and Neurosurgery; Vice Chair for Academic Affairs, Department of Ophthalmology, University of Colorado School of Medicine, Aurora, Colorado

MATTHEW J. THURTELL, MBBS, MSc
Tenured Associate Professor, Department of Ophthalmology and Visual Sciences, University of Iowa Hospitals and Clinics, Iowa City, Iowa

MICHAEL S. VAPHIADES, DO
Departments of Ophthalmology, Neurology and Neurosurgery, University of Alabama at Birmingham, Birmingham, Alabama

MICHAEL WALL, MD
University of Iowa College of Medicine, Veterans Administration Hospital, Iowa City, Iowa

Contents

Preface: Neuro-Ophthalmology for Neurologists xi

Andrew G. Lee

New Treatments for Nonarteritic Anterior Ischemic Optic Neuropathy 1

Rod Foroozan

Despite increasing knowledge about the risk factors and clinical findings of nonarteritic anterior ischemic optic neuropathy (NAION), the treatment of this optic neuropathy has remained limited and without clear evidence-based benefit. Historical treatments of NAION are reviewed, beginning with the Ischemic Optic Neuropathy Decompression Trial. More recent treatments are placed within the historical context and illustrate the need for evidence-based therapy for ischemic optic neuropathy.

Erectile Dysfunction Agents and Nonarteritic Anterior Ischemic Optic Neuropathy 17

Howard D. Pomeranz

Phosphodiesterase-5 inhibitors (PDE5I) are used for treatment of erectile dysfunction and pulmonary arterial hypertension and have been implicated as a causative factor for development of nonarteritic anterior ischemic optic neuropathy (NAION). Controversy remains regarding a cause and effect between PDE5I use and NAION because the mechanism by which NAION occurs is still not well understood. Because neuro-ophthalmologists have accepted that there is a potential relationship between ingestion of the PDE5I class of medications and NAION, the neuro-ophthalmologist should inquire about PDE5I use when evaluating a patient with a new diagnosis of NAION, and counsel patients regarding the implication of continued use of PDE5I.

Homonymous Hemianopia and Vision Restoration Therapy 29

Alexander Frolov, Jeanne Feuerstein, and Prem S. Subramanian

Homonymous hemianopia from stroke causes visual disability. Although some patients experience spontaneous improvement, others have limited to no change and may be left with a severe disability. Current rehabilitation strategies are compensatory and cannot restore function. Animal studies suggest that central nervous system plasticity could allow for redirection of lost visual function into undamaged areas of cortex. A commercial therapy system was developed, from which claims of visual field expansion were disputed by independent researchers. The treatment remains controversial with seemingly contradictory data being generated. Continued research is underway to demonstrate the (non-)efficacy of this treatment method.

Update on Idiopathic Intracranial Hypertension 45

Michael Wall

Idiopathic intracranial hypertension (IIH) is a disorder of elevated intracranial pressure of unknown cause occurring predominantly in young women of childbearing age. The typical patient symptom profile is the presence of

destroy these receptors at the postsynaptic neuromuscular junction. The hallmark of OMG is a history of painless weakness or fatigability of the extraocular muscles and ptosis with normal pupillary function and visual acuity. Clinical, laboratory, electrophysiologic, and pharmacologic tests are available for diagnosis. Treatment can begin with symptom management; there is no cure. Prognosis is improved by use of immunomodulators. Despite advances in treatment, research is needed, especially in the areas of surgical intervention and medical therapy based on risk stratification.

Orbital Disease in Neuro-Ophthalmology **125**

Jessica R. Chang, Anna M. Gruener, and Timothy J. McCulley

Many abnormalities of the orbit present with neuro-ophthalmic findings, such as impaired ocular motility or alignment, and sensory changes, including optic neuropathy. Comprehensive coverage of all orbital diseases is beyond the scope of this article. This review focuses on diagnosis and management of the most common and the most vision- or life-threatening orbital conditions as well as more recently discovered entities and points of active controversy. These conditions include orbital trauma, vascular disease, inflammatory and infectious diseases, and neoplasms. Common presenting symptoms and associated neuro-orbital diseases also are summarized.

The Yield of Diagnostic Imaging in Patients with Isolated Horner Syndrome **145**

Johanna D. Beebe, Randy H. Kardon, and Matthew J. Thurtell

We sought to determine, with a retrospective chart review, the imaging yield for patients with clinically isolated Horner syndrome. MRI/MRA of the head and neck extending from the supraorbital ridge to T4 with fat suppression and with postcontrast images was obtained. Of 88 patients with isolated Horner syndrome who were imaged, 20% had a causative etiology on imaging. The most common cause of an isolated Horner syndrome was a carotid artery dissection. There was 1 patient with a primary malignancy found to be the causative lesion in this group, and 1 patient with spread of their known metastatic disease.

Optical Coherence Tomography in Neuro-ophthalmology **153**

Fiona Costello

The afferent visual pathway is a functionally eloquent region of the central nervous system (CNS). Key clinical features of inflammatory, ischemic, and compressive CNS lesions can be appreciated through detailed ophthalmic examination. Optical coherence tomography (OCT) provides a noninvasive means of capturing manifestations of axonal and neuronal loss in the CNS. OCT represents a surrogate marker of structural integrity in the CNS, through which mechanisms of neurodegeneration and repair may be better understood. In this article, the role of OCT in facilitating the diagnosis and management of several CNS disorders is discussed.

Index **165**

NEUROLOGIC CLINICS

FORTHCOMING ISSUES

May 2017
Dementia
John Ringman, *Editor*

August 2017
Sports Neurology
Tad Seifert, *Editor*

November 2017
Neurocritical Care
Alejandro A. Rabinstein, *Editor*

RECENT ISSUES

November 2016
Global and Domestic Public Health and Neuroepidemiology
David S. Younger, *Editor*

August 2016
Case Studies in Neurology
Randolph W. Evans, *Editor*

May 2016
Optimal Care for Patients with Epilepsy: Practical Aspects
Steven C. Schachter, *Editor*

RELATED INTEREST

Neuroimaging Clinics of North America, August 2015 (Vol. 25, Issue 3)
Orbit and Neuro-ophthalmic Imaging
Juan E. Gutierrez and Bundhit Tantiwongkosi, *Editors*

THE CLINICS ARE AVAILABLE ONLINE!
Access your subscription at:
www.theclinics.com

Preface
Neuro-Ophthalmology for Neurologists

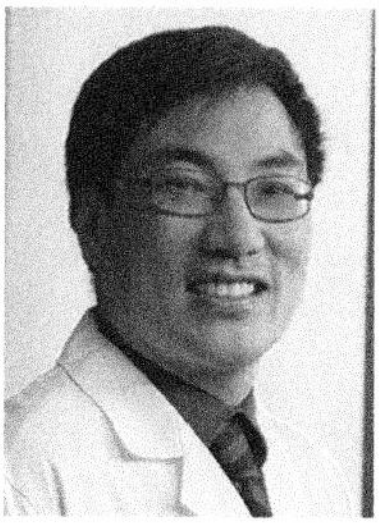

Andrew G. Lee, MD
Editor

In this issue, we discuss several afferent and efferent neuro-ophthalmic conditions of interest to the neurologist. These include new treatments for nonarteritic anterior ischemic optic neuropathy (NAION) and the controversy surrounding erectile dysfunction agents and NAION. In addition, the treatment of homonymous hemianopia with vision restoration and rehabilitation therapy is described. Updates are provided on idiopathic intracranial hypertension (IIH), including the recently completed clinical trial on IIH as well as new information on venous sinus stenting in IIH. Exciting new developments in the management of central retinal artery occlusion and neuromyelitis optica spectrum disorder are discussed. On the efferent side, the difficult clinical and neuroimaging decision making on oculomotor (Third) cranial nerve palsy and ocular myasthenia are described. Finally, orbital disease in neuro-ophthalmology, the evaluation of Horner syndrome, and the utility and future use of optical coherence tomography round out our tour of neuro-ophthalmology.

Andrew G. Lee, MD
Blanton Eye Institute
Houston Methodist Hospital
6560 Fannin Street, Suite 450
Houston, TX 77030, USA

E-mail address:
aglee@houstonmethodist.org

Neurol Clin 35 (2017) xi
http://dx.doi.org/10.1016/j.ncl.2016.09.001
0733-8619/17/© 2016 Published by Elsevier Inc.
neurologic.theclinics.com

New Treatments for Nonarteritic Anterior Ischemic Optic Neuropathy

Rod Foroozan, MD

KEYWORDS

- Ischemic optic neuropathy • Nonarteritic anterior ischemic optic neuropathy (NAION)
- Ischemic Optic Neuropathy Decompression Trial (IONDT)
- Obstructive sleep apnea syndrome (OSAS)

KEY POINTS

- The diagnosis of nonarteritic anterior ischemic optic neuropathy (NAION) is made clinically and without definitive confirmatory ancillary testing.
- The Ischemic Optic Neuropathy Decompression Trial, which showed a lack of benefit of optic nerve sheath decompression, is the largest prospective interventional study of NAION and has helped characterize the natural history of this optic neuropathy.
- Thus far, medical treatment, including with corticosteroids and aspirin, have failed to show a definitive benefit in visual outcomes from NAION.
- Release of vitreopapillary traction may be helpful in some patients who have optic disc edema and visual loss that may resemble NAION.
- The treatment of sleep apnea has been suggested to reduce the risk of fellow eye involvement in patients with NAION.

INTRODUCTION

Nonarteritic anterior ischemic optic neuropathy (NAION) refers to a presumed ischemic process of the anterior portion of the optic nerve. Although many associations with NAION have been reported, none have been proven to be definitively causal. This form of ischemic optic neuropathy has been associated with various risk factors, including advanced age, systemic hypertension, nocturnal hypotension, diabetes mellitus, hyperlipidemia, and a predisposing optic disc morphology.[1,2] A small optic disc and small optic cup have been thought to contribute to a compartment syndrome, which may perpetuate ischemia of the optic disc as axonal swelling develops.[1–3]

Characteristically, NAION presents with a sudden onset of painless visual loss of one eye that may affect visual acuity, visual field, or both, typically in patients older than 50 years.[2] The pupil of the affected eye has a relative afferent pupillary defect

The author reported no conflicts of interest of any portion of the article.
Baylor College of Medicine, 1977 Butler Boulevard, Houston, TX 77030, USA
E-mail address: foroozan@bcm.edu

Neurol Clin 35 (2017) 1–15
http://dx.doi.org/10.1016/j.ncl.2016.08.003

(RAPD), unless there is bilateral and symmetric optic nerve disease. The typical funduscopic appearance acutely includes sectoral or generalized optic disc edema, which may be mildly pale or hyperemic, with associated nerve fiber layer hemorrhage. Acutely, the presence of optic disc edema is required for the diagnosis of NAION (**Fig. 1**), although patients may present later with sector or diffuse optic atrophy. Visual field defects are related to involvement of the nerve fiber bundles as they are anatomically arranged and coalesce to make up the optic disc, and are often altitudinal (**Fig. 2**). The optic disc edema typically lasts weeks and is followed by the development of optic disc pallor and thinning of the involved retinal nerve fiber layer (**Fig. 3**).[4]

Although some forms of ischemic optic neuropathy have a more clearly identifiable cause, for example, with acute severe anemia and hypotension ("shock"),[5] the most common form of this optic neuropathy is spontaneous and idiopathic. This is the form most investigators refer to when discussing NAION and the type that is the basis of this review.

Despite increasing knowledge about the risk factors (**Box 1**) and clinical findings of NAION, the treatment of this optic neuropathy has remained limited and without clear evidence-based benefit. To help understand some of the more recent suggestions, some historical treatments of NAION are reviewed, beginning with the Ischemic Optic Neuropathy Decompression Trial (IONDT). Focusing on treatments since the IONDT, the historical and more recent treatments (**Box 2**) are then blended to help recognize the ongoing frustration in the treatment of this form of ischemic optic neuropathy. Other reviews of the treatment of NAION cover therapies that predated the IONDT.[6,7]

PATHOPHYSIOLOGY AND CLINICAL DIAGNOSIS

NAION is the most common acute optic neuropathy in patients older than 50 years. Ischemia involving the short posterior ciliary arteries (branches of the ophthalmic artery) is the most commonly purported mechanism in NAION.[3] Although optic neuropathy is the mechanism of visual loss, some patients may develop decreased vision because of leakage of fluid within and under the retina.[8] The retinopathy from NAION was likely overlooked more frequently before the routine use of more sensitive imaging techniques, such as optical coherence tomography (OCT) (**Fig. 4**).

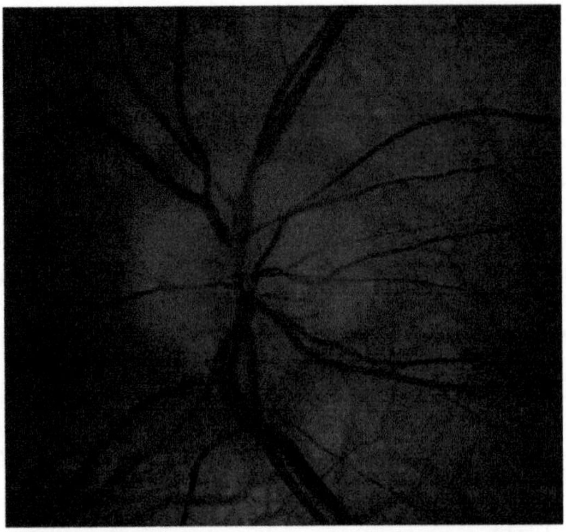

Fig. 1. Fundus photograph of the left eye showing hyperemic optic disc edema in a small optic disc with a small optic disc cup.

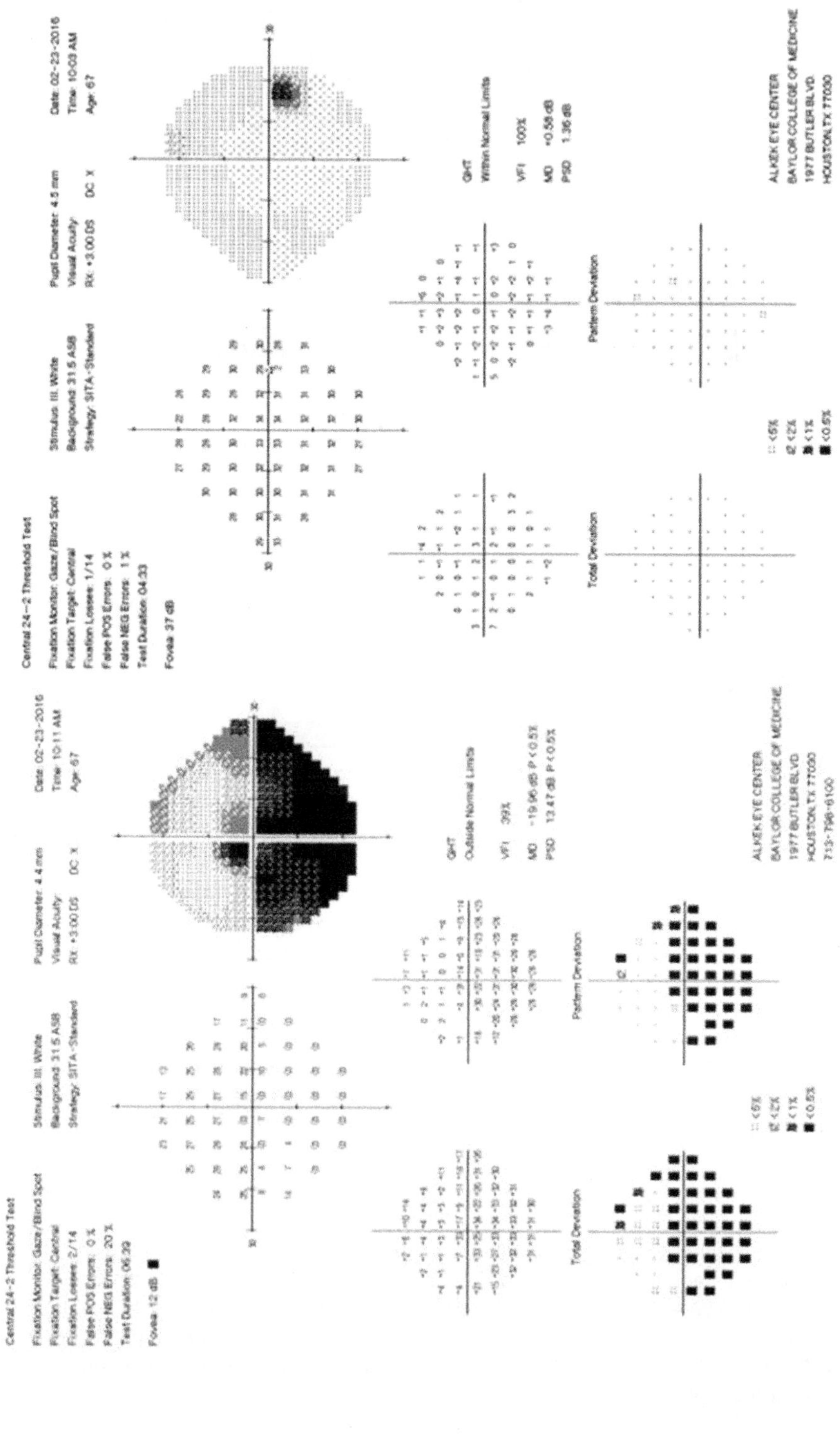

Fig. 2. Automated perimetry showing a full field in the right eye and a central and inferior altitudinal defect in the left eye of a 67-year-old man with NAION.

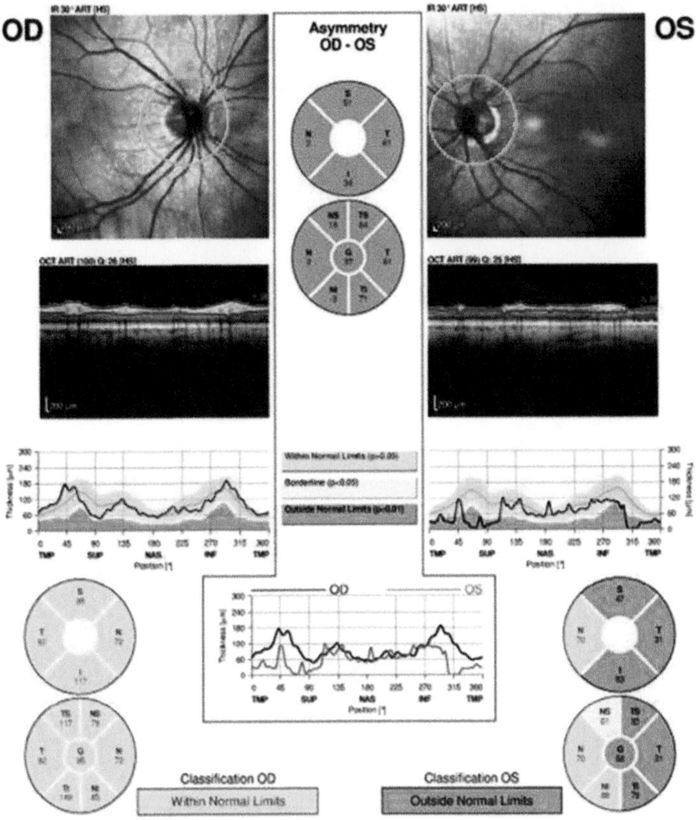

Fig. 3. OCT of the same patient as that in **Fig. 2**, showing decreased retinal nerve fiber layer measures superiorly and temporally in the left eye after resolution of optic disc edema from NAION. The measures of the right eye were normal.

Part of the difficulty with NAION is the lack of a confirmatory test to prove that the diagnosis is correct. In contrast to inflammatory or demyelinating optic neuritis, cranial and orbital MRI with contrast typically shows no evidence of optic nerve enhancement.[9] Blood tests are often performed to exclude other causes of optic disc edema, such as arteritic anterior ischemic optic neuropathy (eg, erythrocyte sedimentation rate) or inflammatory optic neuropathy. NAION has remained a clinical diagnosis and no one test can be done to prove that one is dealing with this type of optic neuropathy; ancillary testing can be done only to show what it is not.

Helping to confuse the issue is the lack of consistent parallel of NAION with intracranial stroke or retinal arterial occlusion. In NAION there is

- No consistent increase in white matter changes suggestive of ischemic stroke on neuroimaging[10]
- No consistent link to carotid occlusive disease[11]
- No consistent link to increased risk of cardiac or cerebrovascular disease[12]
- No definitive evidence that treatment of underlying vascular risk factors alters the course of the acute optic neuropathy or reduces the risk of fellow eye involvement
- A low rate (around 5%) of recurrence of ischemic optic neuropathy in an initially affected eye

Box 1
Suggested associated systemic risk factors in nonarteritic anterior ischemic optic neuropathy

Hypertension

Diabetes mellitus

Nocturnal hypotension

Obstructive sleep apnea syndrome

Hyperlipidemia

Smoking

Data from Biousse V, Newman NJ. Ischemic optic neuropathies. N Engl J Med 2015;372:2428–36; Miller NR, Arnold AC. Current concepts in the diagnosis, pathogenesis and management of nonarteritic anterior ischaemic optic neuropathy. Eye (Lond) 2015;29:65–79.

Despite this, NAION is frequently referred to as a "stroke" of the optic nerve when the diagnosis is discussed with patients. Even arterial insufficiency as the underlying pathophysiology of NAION has been repeatedly questioned and some have suggested it may be a venous rather than arterial disease.[13]

Box 2
Summary of treatments attempted for nonarteritic anterior ischemic optic neuropathy by route of administration

Surgical

Optic nerve sheath decompression

Radial optic neurotomy

Vitrectomy with relief of vitreous traction

Topical

Brimonidine

Intravitreal

Corticosteroids

Anti–vascular endothelial growth factor agents

Other

Systemic

Corticosteroids

Levodopa

Aspirin

Treatment of obstructive sleep apnea

Pheresis

Other

Transcorneal electrical stimulation

Vision restoration therapy

Acupuncture

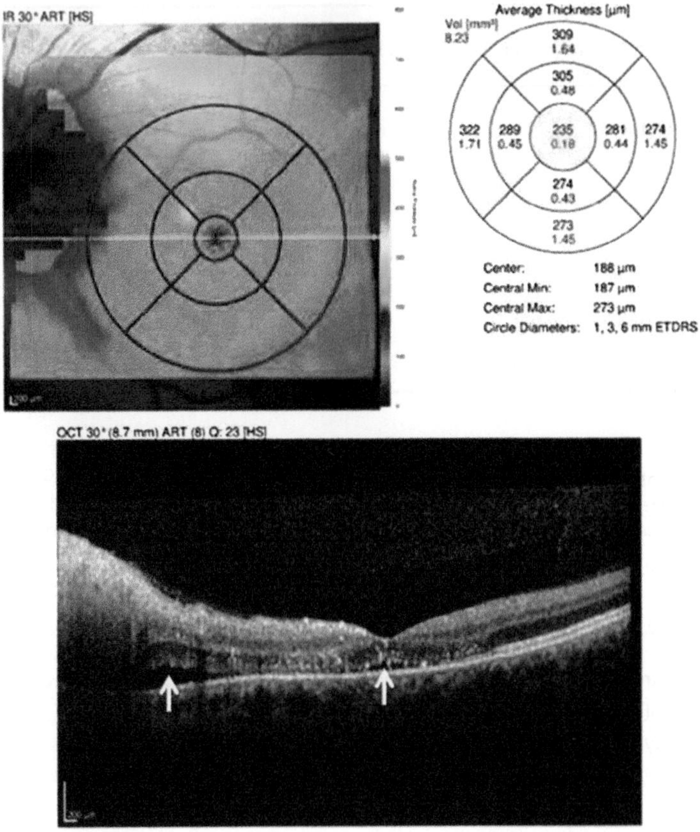

Fig. 4. OCT showing macular thickening and subretinal fluid (*arrows*) in the left eye of a patient with optic disc edema from NAION.

Some investigators have questioned the role of the vitreous in contributing or causing NAION.[14] Although the significance of vitreous traction in typical NAION is not clear, some patients develop more chronic optic disc edema from a tractional effect of the overlying vitreous and progressive visual loss may result from it (**Fig. 5**).

Finally, evidence of clinicopathologic correlation in NAION is limited. A frequently cited example of the pathology of acute NAION was confounded by anemia requiring 4 units of packed red blood cells days before the onset of visual loss.[15]

ISCHEMIC OPTIC NEUROPATHY DECOMPRESSION TRIAL

In the 1980s, there was increasing evidence to suggest that creating a surgical opening in the optic nerve sheath could improve visual function in patients with NAION,[16] potentially by limiting the extent of ischemia created by the compartment syndrome contributed to by a small optic disc and cup. The IONDT was a prospective, multicenter, randomized, controlled trial designed to assess the safety and efficacy of optic nerve decompression surgery (ONDS) compared with observation in patients with NAION.[17] The study contributed to much of what is understood of the natural history of disease.[18]

The eligibility requirements of the IONDT included a sudden onset of visual loss, best-corrected visual acuity of 20/64 or worse in the affected eye, an RAPD (bilateral

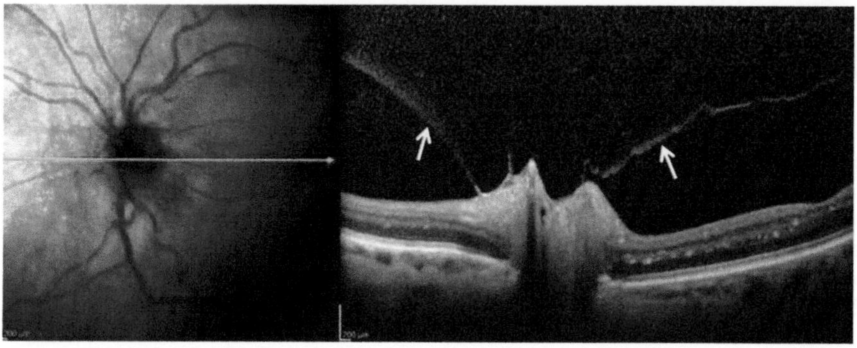

Fig. 5. OCT of the left eye showing optic disc elevation and hyperreflectivity consistent with vitreous (*arrows*) resulting in traction on the nerve head.

disease excepted), optic disc edema, and a visual field defect consistent with an optic neuropathy. Patients were 50 years of age or older and the duration of symptoms was fewer than 14 days at the time of enrollment. Patients were excluded if they had clinical features that suggested a disorder other than NAION, such as an elevated erythrocyte sedimentation rate or a history of inflammatory disease. They were also excluded if they had no light perception vision, sequential NAION within 14 days, a condition that increased their surgical risk, or an ophthalmologic condition that would confound assessment of visual function.

Patients whose exclusion was based solely on visual acuity that was too good to enter the study were allowed to participate if their vision deteriorated to 20/64 or worse within 30 days from the onset of symptoms. This group was referred to as the late-entry group. Patients who satisfied the inclusion criteria were randomized into the ONDS group or the observation group. Patients whose visual acuity remained better than 20/64 were followed and their natural history was observed.

The study began in October 1992 and the randomization was concluded in October 1994 on recommendation of the Data and Safety Monitoring Committee. The preliminary data were made available in 1995 and the complete data in 1996. A total of 1680 patients were screened and 420 patients were diagnosed with NAION. Of these 420 patients, 207 (49%) had a baseline examination visual acuity better than 20/64 and 213 (51%) had a visual acuity of 20/64 or worse. From this group of 420 patients with NAION, 258 patients met the visual acuity requirement, either as a regular entry (213 patients) or as a late entry (45 patients). These 258 patients were randomized either to surgery or observation. Of the 162 remaining patients who were not randomized, 148 patients maintained a visual acuity better than 20/64 over a 30-day period. Of the 14 remaining patients whose visual acuity was 20/64 or worse, 12 patients refused randomization and 2 patients were not offered randomization because of a breach in protocol. Although these 162 patients were not randomized, they were followed to observe the natural history of the optic neuropathy.

The IONDT showed that patients who had surgery did no better when compared with patients assigned to careful follow-up regarding improved visual acuity of 3 or more lines at 6 months: 32.6% of the surgery group improved compared with 42.7% of the observation group. In addition, patients who had surgery had a significantly greater risk of losing 3 or more lines of vision at 6 months: 23.9% in the surgery group worsened compared with 12.4% in the observation group.

The results of the IONDT suggested that ONDS for NAION was not effective and may be harmful. The IONDT Research Group recommended that ONDS not be performed for NAION.

Previous NAION or other optic neuropathy was present in the fellow eye of 88 (21.1%) of 418 patients at baseline. Four patients developed optic neuropathy in the fellow eye at follow-up that could not be conclusively diagnosed as NAION. New NAION in the fellow eye occurred in 48 (14.7%) of 326 patients at risk during a median follow-up of 5.1 years.[18,19] Other reports have documented even higher rates of sequential NAION, with some as high as 40%; however, 1 large series of 431 patients found that the 2-year cumulative probability of developing NAION in the fellow eye was 15% and 20% at 5 years.[20]

SURGICAL THERAPY

A different approach to the theoretic risk from the compartment syndrome caused by ischemia involving a small optic disc and cup was to relax the scleral ring from an intraocular approach. Transvitreal optic neurotomy was performed in 7 eyes of 7 patients with NAION.[21] An average of 10 lines of visual improvement was noted. The study was not randomized and not masked and the investigators suggested a randomized clinical trial. Little has been published on radial optic neuropathy since this appeared in 2003.

Visual improvement from release of vitreous traction through vitrectomy has been suggested by some investigators. In 15 (94%) of 16 patients with NAION, visual acuity improved and 9 eyes (56%) had an improvement of 3 or more lines of visual acuity[22]; however, other investigators have called into question the OCT images depicting vitreous traction in this study, and the role of vitreous traction in all patients with NAION.[23] Some patients with optic disc edema from vitreopapillary traction syndrome may be mistaken to have NAION. In that subgroup of patients with progressive optic disc edema and visual loss, release of the vitreous traction on the optic disc by vitrectomy can be helpful.[24]

To summarize the outcomes of surgical treatment of NAION, a Cochrane review published in 2015 found only 1 trial (the IONDT) met criteria for the review. All the other studies were nonrandomized or uncontrolled.[25]

TOPICAL

Brimonidine, an alpha agonist frequently used as a topical agent for glaucoma, has been purported to have a neuroprotective effect, particularly in animal studies. A randomized controlled trial in Europe enrolled 36 patients (eventually 18 received placebo and 11 brimonidine and all received aspirin) with NAION and symptoms of 7 days' duration or less.[26] The planned sample size of 132 patients could not be achieved, most commonly because of delay in presentation beyond 7 days. There was no statistically significant benefit of brimonidine in any of the visual function outcomes measured when compared with placebo.

INTRAVITREAL

Intravitreal injections have become some of the most common procedures in ophthalmology and are often performed for age-related macular degeneration (ARMD) and retinal vascular occlusive disease. This route provides more directed therapy and helps limit the systemic side effects of the injected substance. Corticosteroids, most commonly intravitreal triamcinolone acetonide (IVTA), have been injected into the vitreous with hopes that they will help resolve the optic disc edema. The studies have been without randomization and results have been mixed.[27,28] In a group of 36 patients with NAION, an improvement in visual acuity at 6 months was noted in patients treated with IVTA.[29] In the treated group, there was a significant inverse correlation between the delay of the injection and the visual acuity achieved at 6 months ($P<.0083$, $r = -0.56$). A significant improvement of the visual field was noted in the injected group when compared with the nontreated group at 6 months ($P<.0028$). Longer-acting steroids, in the form of an intravitreal dexamethasone implant, did not alter visual function in 3 patients with NAION.[30]

The proliferation of the use of anti–vascular endothelial growth factor (VEGF) agents for ARMD and retinal vascular occlusive disease helped spur interest in their use for NAION.[31] In a nonrandomized trial, intravitreal injection of bevacizumab was performed in 17 patients with NAION, and when compared with 8 controls there was no difference in measures of visual function or structural measures of the optic nerve by OCT.[32] Unfortunately, in a rodent[33] and nonhuman primate model of NAION,[34] ranibizumab did not affect the ensuing optic nerve damage.

Intravitreal injection has provided a route for a number of other substances that have been explored in animal models and in humans with NAION. These have included aflibercept,[35] ciliary neurotrophic factor,[36] prostaglandin J2,[37] fasudil (a Rho-kinase inhibitor),[38] and erythropoietin.[39] The studies have all been preliminary, in a small number of subjects, and have not yet produced conclusive evidence of efficacy.

SYSTEMIC

Corticosteroids

A theoretic basis for the use of corticosteroids in anterior ischemic optic neuropathy focused on the potential benefits of hastening the resolution of optic disc edema. Although corticosteroids had been used in NAION, even before the results of the IONDT were published, there was renewed interest after the results of a large series of patients were published in 2008. From 1973 to 2000 a cohort of 613 patients with NAION was followed, and 312 patients voluntarily opted for corticosteroids, 80 mg of prednisone for 2 weeks, followed by a tapering course over the ensuing several weeks.[40] At 6 months from the onset of NAION, of the eyes with initial visual acuity 20/70 or worse and seen within 2 weeks of onset, there was visual acuity improvement in 69.8% (95% confidence interval [CI] 57.3%–79.9%) in the treated group, compared with 40.5% (95% CI 29.2%–52.9%) in the untreated group (odds ratio of improvement: 3.39; 95% CI 1.62–7.11; $P = .001$). This study suggested that eyes with NAION treated during the acute phase with systemic corticosteroids had a significantly higher probability of improvement in visual acuity ($P = .001$) and visual field ($P = .005$) than in the untreated group. The study was not randomized and was not masked, but despite this, did rekindle the discussion, including the potential benefit of improving macular edema, of the use of corticosteroids for NAION.[41] Since then, a lack of benefit of corticosteroids (80 mg of oral prednisolone[42] and intravenous methylprednisolone 1 g per day[43] as given in the Optic Neuritis Treatment Trial), initiated within 2 weeks of the onset of visual symptoms, has been noted by 2 other groups.

A prospective randomized trial from Germany of fluocortolone (a glucocorticoid more commonly used topically in the United States) and pentoxifylline versus pentoxifylline alone showed that patients treated with steroids were more likely to experience an improvement and less likely to have a worsening of visual acuity.[44] Thirty patients were "quasi-randomized" in each group within 3 days (earlier than prior successfully completed intervention studies of NAION) of loss of visual acuity. Visual acuity was remeasured at 3 days and 6 months after the onset of treatment. Although visual acuity was statistically improved in patients treated with steroids, there was no statistically significant improvement in visual fields. Enrollment based on symptomatic loss of acuity may have biased the patients in this study as early on patients with NAION may recognize loss of visual field before loss of central vision ensues. There was no notation of whether any studies were done to assess for macular edema, and the use of pentoxifylline in both groups makes the data more difficult to interpret in the context of the natural history of NAION.

Levodopa

The efficacy of levodopa for NAION was purported after 1 study found that patients treated with levodopa within 45 days of the onset of symptoms were more likely to have an improvement and less likely to have worsening of visual acuity as compared with untreated patients.[45] However, the statistical methods and the validity of the results were questioned.[46–49] A follow-up study published in 2015 assessed 59 patients with NAION seen within 15 days of the onset of visual loss. All patients were offered levodopa (25 mg carbidopa/100 mg levodopa 3 times daily for 12 weeks). This was a self-selection study and patients who took levodopa had worse visual function at onset. Patients with 20/60 or worse initial visual acuity treated with levodopa had significant improvement ($P<.0001$) in the mean change from initial to final logMAR visual acuity, whereas the mean change for the control group was not significant ($P = .23$). In the levodopa group 19 (83%) of 23 patients improved and none got worse, as compared with 6 (43%) of 14 in the control group who improved and 4 (29%) worsened. It was curious that the change in visual field mean deviation and retinal nerve fiber layer thickness on OCT (assessment of the macula was not done) showed no significant difference between the 2 groups. As perimetry and retinal nerve fiber measurements should theoretically improve in tandem with improvements in visual acuity, it is difficult to reconcile the benefits on acuity alone in this study. My experience has been, despite statistically significant evidence of benefit, levodopa is an infrequently used treatment in NAION.

Aspirin

Given the relative frequency of fellow eye involvement, some investigators have attempted therapeutic intervention aimed at the prevention of sequential NAION.[50] A new diagnosis of NAION was not found to be affected by aspirin in the IONDT.[19] To assess the efficacy of aspirin therapy in preventing sequential NAION, a retrospective cohort study of 431 patients with unilateral NAION was conducted.[20] Following the development of NAION, 153 patients were prescribed and 278 were not prescribed aspirin. The investigators found that the 2-year cumulative probability of sequential NAION was 7% in the aspirin group and 15% in the nonaspirin group, and the 5-year cumulative probabilities were 17% and 20%, respectively. They suggested that aspirin may have a short-term benefit but did not offer long-term protection. Despite the lack of epidemiologic support, my experience has been that aspirin, anticoagulants, and anti-platelet agents are frequently suggested to patients who have had NAION not only by ophthalmologists but by neurologists and internists.

Treatment of Sleep Apnea

Obstructive sleep apnea syndrome (OSAS) has been associated with NAION.[51] The degree of the association has varied, in part depending on the criteria used for the diagnosis of OSAS. A meta-analysis of 4 prospective cohort studies and one case-control study found that the pooled odds ratio of developing NAION in patients with OSAS was 6.18 (95% CI 2.00–19.11) versus non-OSAS controls.[52] In a cohort study of 89 patients with NAION, all patients underwent polysomnography to diagnose

OSAS and were prospectively followed to determine the rate of second eye involvement. Sixty-seven (75%) patients had OSAS and fellow eye involvement was noted in 10 (13.7%) of 73 patients at 3 years.[53] The fellow eye developed NAION in 8 (15.4%) of 52 patients with OSAS and 2 (9.5%) of 21 patients without OSAS (P = .04). The risk of fellow eye involvement was significantly greater (hazard ratio 5.54; 95% CI 1.13–27.11; P = .04) in patients with severe OSAS (apnea-hypopnea index $\geq$ 30) who did not adhere to the treatment with continuous positive airway pressure (CPAP). The overall rate of second eye involvement (13.7%) at 3 years was similar to that of the IONDT (14.7%) at 5 years. The lack of randomization limits the generalizability of the study, and although the treatment of OSAS with CPAP may lower the risk of subsequent NAION it has not been preventative.[54]

Apheresis

A group from Italy suggested low-density lipoprotein apheresis (LA) could improve visual outcomes in NAION[55]; however, in a series of 10 patients treated with LA there was no difference in visual function after 6 months when compared with 10 patients treated with "conventional" therapy.[56]

Other

Transcorneal electrical stimulation (TES) via corneal electrodes has been purported to improve visual acuity in patients with NAION and, in the same study, traumatic optic neuropathy.[57] The proposed mechanism of action was a neuroprotective effect of electrical stimulation and TES was said to be neuroprotective in a rodent model of NAION.[58]

Visual restoration therapy has been said to lead to functional improvement in patients with visual deficits including homonymous hemianopia and optic neuropathy.[59] A randomized study of 10 patients with stable visual loss from NAION showed a limited effect on visual function, including reading speed.[60]

Acupuncture has been said to be helpful for optic neuropathy, although a Cochrane review published in 2013 was not able to draw any conclusions about its effect in treating glaucoma.[61] A group from China noted that in 69 patients (and 93 affected eyes) with NAION, acupuncture could "obviously improve the visual function of patients with NAION."[62] Nine (13%) of the 69 patients had simultaneous NAION and there was no control group.

SUMMARY

Although understanding of some clinical findings and risk factors has improved, there remains no definitive proven treatment for NAION. A review of the treatments attempted highlights the importance of clinical trials and the impact of randomization. As of March 2016 there were 21 trials focused on anterior ischemic optic neuropathy (www.clinicaltrials.gov; search ischemic optic neuropathy). Twelve were completed or withdrawn and 4 were recruiting patients. There is hope that animal models will provide insight into the pathophysiology and new avenues for treatment of this optic neuropathy. We are hopeful that novel treatments may alter the course of the acute optic neuropathy and diminish the risk of fellow eye involvement. My sense is that before we get there clinical trials will need to reassess some longstanding beliefs and address unanswered questions in order to:

- Provide more concrete confirmation of the diagnosis of NAION
- Assess the potential association between NAION and central nervous ischemia
- Assess the impact of treatment of proposed systemic vascular risk factors and their effect on fellow eye involvement

Box 3
Suggestions for prospective studies of treatment of nonarteritic anterior ischemic optic neuropathy

- Be randomized and controlled
- Include a thorough assessment of optic nerve function, including more than visual acuity
- Include ancillary studies of optic nerve and optic disc structure (retinal nerve fiber layer and ganglion cell layer)
- Include structural assessment (optical coherence tomography) of the macula and account for the role of maculopathy

Based on this review of the failed treatments thus far some suggestions for new studies can be made (**Box 3**). Eventually randomized, controlled trials will most likely be needed to help a putative new therapy become standard of care.

REFERENCES

1. Biousse V, Newman NJ. Ischemic optic neuropathies. N Engl J Med 2015;372: 2428–36.
2. Miller NR, Arnold AC. Current concepts in the diagnosis, pathogenesis and management of nonarteritic anterior ischaemic optic neuropathy. Eye (Lond) 2015;29: 65–79.
3. Arnold AC. Pathogenesis of nonarteritic anterior ischemic optic neuropathy. J Neuroophthalmol 2003;23:157–63.
4. Akbari M, Abdi P, Fard MA, et al. Retinal ganglion cell loss precedes retinal nerve fiber thinning in nonarteritic anterior ischemic optic neuropathy. J Neuroophthalmol 2016;36(2):141–6.
5. Foroozan R, Buono LM, Savino PJ. Optic disc structure and shock-induced anterior ischemic optic neuropathy. Ophthalmology 2003;110:327–31.
6. Atkins EJ, Bruce BB, Newman NJ, et al. Treatment of nonarteritic anterior ischemic optic neuropathy. Surv Ophthalmol 2010;55:47–63.
7. Katz DM, Trobe JD. Is there treatment for nonarteritic anterior ischemic optic neuropathy. Curr Opin Ophthalmol 2015;26:458–63.
8. Hedges TR 3rd, Vuong LN, Gonzalez-Garcia AO, et al. Subretinal fluid from anterior ischemic optic neuropathy demonstrated by optical coherence tomography. Arch Ophthalmol 2008;126:812–5.
9. Rizzo JF 3rd, Andreoli CM, Rabinov JD. Use of magnetic resonance imaging to differentiate optic neuritis and nonarteritic anterior ischemic optic neuropathy. Ophthalmology 2002;109:1679–84.
10. Deramo VA, Sergott RC, Augsburger JJ, et al. Ischemic optic neuropathy as the first manifestation of elevated cholesterol levels in young patients. Ophthalmology 2003;110:1041–6 [discussion: 1046].
11. Fry CL, Carter JE, Kanter MC, et al. Anterior ischemic optic neuropathy is not associated with carotid artery atherosclerosis. Stroke 1993;24:539–42.
12. Hasanreisoglu M, Robenshtok E, Ezrahi D, et al. Do patients with non-arteritic ischemic optic neuritis have increased risk for cardiovascular and cerebrovascular events? Neuroepidemiology 2013;40:220–4.
13. Levin LA, Danesh-Meyer HV. Hypothesis: a venous etiology for nonarteritic anterior ischemic optic neuropathy. Arch Ophthalmol 2008;126:1582–5.

14. Parsa CF, Hoyt WF. Nonarteritic anterior ischemic optic neuropathy (NAION): a misnomer. Rearranging pieces of a puzzle to reveal a nonischemic papillopathy caused by vitreous separation. Ophthalmology 2015;122:439–42.
15. Tesser RA, Niendorf ER, Levin LA. The morphology of an infarct in nonarteritic anterior ischemic optic neuropathy. Ophthalmology 2003;110:2031–5.
16. Sergott RC, Cohen MS, Bosley TM, et al. Optic nerve decompression may improve the progressive form of nonarteritic ischemic optic neuropathy. Arch Ophthalmol 1989;107:1743–54.
17. Optic nerve decompression surgery for nonarteritic anterior ischemic optic neuropathy (NAION) is not effective and may be harmful. The Ischemic Optic Neuropathy Decompression Trial Research Group. JAMA 1995;273:625–32.
18. Characteristics of patients with nonarteritic anterior ischemic optic neuropathy eligible for the Ischemic Optic Neuropathy Decompression Trial. Arch Ophthalmol 1996;114:1366–74.
19. Newman NJ, Scherer R, Langenberg P, et al. The fellow eye in NAION: report from the ischemic optic neuropathy decompression trial follow-up study. Am J Ophthalmol 2002;134:317–28.
20. Beck RW, Hayreh SS, Podhajsky PA, et al. Aspirin therapy in nonarteritic anterior ischemic optic neuropathy. Am J Ophthalmol 1997;123:212–7.
21. Soheilian M, Koochek A, Yazdani S, et al. Transvitreal optic neurotomy for nonarteritic anterior ischemic optic neuropathy. Retina 2003;23:692–7.
22. Modarres M, Sanjari MS, Falavarjani KG. Vitrectomy and release of presumed epipapillary vitreous traction for treatment of nonarteritic anterior ischemic optic neuropathy associated with partial posterior vitreous detachment. Ophthalmology 2007;114:340–4.
23. Lee MS, Foroozan R, Kosmorsky GS. Posterior vitreous detachment in AION. Ophthalmology 2009;116:597–597.e1.
24. Meyer CH, Schmidt JC, Mennel S, et al. Functional and anatomical results of vitreopapillary traction after vitrectomy. Acta Ophthalmol Scand 2007;85:221–2.
25. Dickersin K, Li T. Surgery for nonarteritic anterior ischemic optic neuropathy. Cochrane Database Syst Rev 2015;(3):CD001538.
26. Wilhelm B, Ludtke H, Wilhelm H. Efficacy and tolerability of 0.2% brimonidine tartrate for the treatment of acute non-arteritic anterior ischemic optic neuropathy (NAION): a 3-month, double-masked, randomised, placebo-controlled trial. Graefes Arch Clin Exp Ophthalmol 2006;244:551–8.
27. Jonas JB, Spandau UH, Harder B, et al. Intravitreal triamcinolone acetonide for treatment of acute nonarteritic anterior ischemic optic neuropathy. Graefes Arch Clin Exp Ophthalmol 2007;245:749–50.
28. Kaderli B, Avci R, Yucel A, et al. Intravitreal triamcinolone improves recovery of visual acuity in nonarteritic anterior ischemic optic neuropathy. J Neuroophthalmol 2007;27:164–8.
29. Radoi C, Garcia T, Brugniart C, et al. Intravitreal triamcinolone injections in nonarteritic anterior ischemic optic neuropathy. Graefes Arch Clin Exp Ophthalmol 2014;252:339–45.
30. Alten F, Clemens CR, Heiduschka P, et al. Intravitreal dexamethasone implant [Ozurdex] for the treatment of nonarteritic anterior ischemic optic neuropathy. Doc Ophthalmol 2014;129:203–7.
31. Prescott CR, Sklar CA, Lesser RL, et al. Is intravitreal bevacizumab an effective treatment option for nonarteritic anterior ischemic optic neuropathy? J Neuroophthalmol 2012;32:51–3.

32. Rootman DB, Gill HS, Margolin EA. Intravitreal bevacizumab for the treatment of nonarteritic anterior ischemic optic neuropathy: a prospective trial. Eye (Lond) 2013;27:538–44.
33. Huang TL, Chang CH, Chang SW, et al. Efficacy of intravitreal injections of anti-vascular endothelial growth factor agents in a rat model of anterior ischemic optic neuropathy. Invest Ophthalmol Vis Sci 2015;56:2290–6.
34. Miller NR, Johnson MA, Nolan T, et al. A single intravitreal injection of ranibizumab provides no neuroprotection in a nonhuman primate model of moderate-to-severe nonarteritic anterior ischemic optic neuropathy. Invest Ophthalmol Vis Sci 2015; 56:7679–86.
35. Ayhan Z, Kocaoglu G, Yaman A, et al. Single intravitreal aflibercept injection for unilateral acute nonarteritic ischemic optic neuropathy. Case Rep Ophthalmol Med 2015;2015:783241.
36. Mathews MK, Guo Y, Langenberg P, et al. Ciliary neurotrophic factor (CNTF)-mediated ganglion cell survival in a rodent model of non-arteritic anterior ischaemic optic neuropathy (NAION). Br J Ophthalmol 2015;99:133–7.
37. Miller NR, Johnson MA, Nolan T, et al. Sustained neuroprotection from a single intravitreal injection of PGJ(2) in a nonhuman primate model of nonarteritic anterior ischemic optic neuropathy. Invest Ophthalmol Vis Sci 2014;55:7047–56.
38. Sanjari N, Pakravan M, Nourinia R, et al. Intravitreal injection of a Rho-kinase inhibitor (fasudil) for recent onset non-arteritic anterior ischemic optic neuropathy. J Clin Pharmacol 2015;56(6):749–53.
39. Modarres M, Falavarjani KG, Nazari H, et al. Intravitreal erythropoietin injection for the treatment of non-arteritic anterior ischaemic optic neuropathy. Br J Ophthalmol 2011;95:992–5.
40. Hayreh SS, Zimmerman MB. Non-arteritic anterior ischemic optic neuropathy: role of systemic corticosteroid therapy. Graefes Arch Clin Exp Ophthalmol 2008;246:1029–46.
41. Lee AG, Biousse V. Should steroids be offered to patients with nonarteritic anterior ischemic optic neuropathy? J Neuroophthalmol 2010;30:193–8.
42. Rebolleda G, Perez-Lopez M, Casas LP, et al. Visual and anatomical outcomes of non-arteritic anterior ischemic optic neuropathy with high-dose systemic corticosteroids. Graefes Arch Clin Exp Ophthalmol 2013;251:255–60.
43. Kinori M, Ben-Bassat I, Wasserzug Y, et al. Visual outcome of mega-dose intravenous corticosteroid treatment in non-arteritic anterior ischemic optic neuropathy—retrospective analysis. BMC Ophthalmol 2014;14:62.
44. Prokosch V, Thanos S. Visual outcome of patients following NAION after treatment with adjunctive fluocortolone. Restor Neurol Neurosci 2014;32:381–9.
45. Johnson LN, Guy ME, Krohel GB, et al. Levodopa may improve vision loss in recent-onset, nonarteritic anterior ischemic optic neuropathy. Ophthalmology 2000;107:521–6.
46. Cox TA. Does levodopa improve visual function in NAION? Ophthalmology 2000; 107:1431.
47. Johnson LN, Madsen RW, Krohel GB. Author's reply. Ophthalmology 2000;107: 1431.
48. Beck RW. Does Levodopa improve visual function in NAION? Ophthalmology 2000;107:1431–4 [discusson: 1435–8].
49. Hayreh SS. Does Levodopa improve visual function in NAION? Ophthalmology 2000;107:1434–8.

50. Salomon O, Huna-Baron R, Steinberg DM, et al. Role of aspirin in reducing the frequency of second eye involvement in patients with non-arteritic anterior ischaemic optic neuropathy. Eye (Lond) 1999;13(Pt 3a):357–9.
51. Mojon DS, Hedges TR 3rd, Ehrenberg B, et al. Association between sleep apnea syndrome and nonarteritic anterior ischemic optic neuropathy. Arch Ophthalmol 2002;120:601–5.
52. Wu Y, Zhou LM, Lou H, et al. The association between obstructive sleep apnea and nonarteritic anterior ischemic optic neuropathy: a systematic review and meta-analysis. Curr Eye Res 2016;41(7):987–92.
53. Aptel F, Khayi H, Pepin JL, et al. Association of nonarteritic ischemic optic neuropathy with obstructive sleep apnea syndrome: consequences for obstructive sleep apnea screening and treatment. JAMA Ophthalmol 2015;133:797–804.
54. Behbehani R, Mathews MK, Sergott RC, et al. Nonarteritic anterior ischemic optic neuropathy in patients with sleep apnea while being treated with continuous positive airway pressure. Am J Ophthalmol 2005;139:518–21.
55. Ramunni A, Giancipoli G, Saracino A, et al. LDL-apheresis in acute anterior ischemic optic neuropathy. Int J Artif Organs 2004;27:337–41.
56. Guerriero S, Giancipoli G, Cantatore A, et al. LDL apheresis in the treatment of non-arteritic ischaemic optic neuropathy: a 6-month follow-up study. Eye (Lond) 2009;23:1343–4.
57. Fujikado T, Morimoto T, Matsushita K, et al. Effect of transcorneal electrical stimulation in patients with nonarteritic ischemic optic neuropathy or traumatic optic neuropathy. Jpn J Ophthalmol 2006;50:266–73.
58. Osako T, Chuman H, Maekubo T, et al. Effects of steroid administration and transcorneal electrical stimulation on the anatomic and electrophysiologic deterioration of nonarteritic ischemic optic neuropathy in a rodent model. Jpn J Ophthalmol 2013;57:410–5.
59. Mueller I, Mast H, Sabel BA. Recovery of visual field defects: a large clinical observational study using vision restoration therapy. Restor Neurol Neurosci 2007;25:563–72.
60. Jung CS, Bruce B, Newman NJ, et al. Visual function in anterior ischemic optic neuropathy: effect of Vision Restoration Therapy–a pilot study. J Neurol Sci 2008;268:145–9.
61. Law SK, Li T. Acupuncture for glaucoma. Cochrane Database Syst Rev 2013;(5):CD006030.
62. Qin Y, Yuan W, Deng H, et al. Clinical efficacy observation of acupuncture treatment for nonarteritic anterior ischemic optic neuropathy. Evid Based Complement Alternat Med 2015;2015:713218.

Erectile Dysfunction Agents and Nonarteritic Anterior Ischemic Optic Neuropathy

Howard D. Pomeranz, MD, PhD

KEYWORDS

• Erectile dysfunction drug • Non-arteritic anterior ischemic optic neuropathy
• Phosphodiesterase 5 inhibitor • Pfizer • Sildenafil • Tadalafil • Vardenafil

KEY POINTS

- Phosphodiesterase-5 inhibitors (PDE5I) are used for treatment of erectile dysfunction and pulmonary arterial hypertension.
- PDE5Is have been implicated in being a causative factor for development of nonarteritic anterior ischemic optic neuropathy (NAION).
- The relationship between PDE5I and NAION has been based on the publication of case reports that have documented loss of vision due to NAION after ingestion of sildenafil or tadalafil.
- A case-crossover study has shown a twofold risk of developing NAION within 1 day after use of PDE5I.
- Neuro-ophthalmologists have accepted that there is a potential relationship and inquire about PDE5I use when evaluating a patient with a new diagnosis of NAION.

INTRODUCTION

Phosphodiesterase-5 inhibitors (PDE5I), which are used for treatment of erectile dysfunction (ED) and pulmonary arterial hypertension, have been implicated in being a causative factor for development of nonarteritic anterior ischemic optic neuropathy (NAION). The relationship between PDE5I and NAION has been based on the publication of case reports that have documented loss of vision due to NAION after ingestion of sildenafil or tadalafil starting in 2000, but more recently has been supported by a case-crossover retrospective study. There still remains controversy regarding a cause-and-effect relationship between PDE5I and NAION. The mechanism by which

No funding support.
The author has nothing to disclose.
Department of Ophthalmology, Northwell Health, 600 Northern Boulevard, Suite 214, Great Neck, NY 11021, USA
E-mail address: hpomeran@northwell.edu

Neurol Clin 35 (2017) 17–27
http://dx.doi.org/10.1016/j.ncl.2016.08.007

NAION occurs is still not well understood. This raises doubts about its potential relationship with PDE5I because one must explain how this class of medications has its effect on circulation to the optic nerve in a situation in which the pathophysiology of NAION itself is not known. Nonetheless, neuro-ophthalmologists have accepted that there is a potential relationship and inquire about PDE5I use when evaluating a patient with a new diagnosis of NAION.

History of Erectile Dysfunction Drug Development and Mechanism of Action

The PDE5Is that are approved by the Food and Drug Administration (FDA) include the following:

- Sildenafil
- Vardenafil
- Tadalafil
- Avanafil

Sildenafil was first synthesized by pharmaceutical chemists working at Pfizer and was initially studied for use in treatment of hypertension and angina. Phase I clinical trials suggested that the drug had little effect on angina but could induce penile erection.

The FDA approved these medications for treatment of ED as follows:

- Sildenafil (Viagra) in March 1998
- Vardenafil (Levitra) in August 2003
- Tadalafil (Cialis) in November 2003
- Avanafil (Stendra) in April 2012

Udenafil (Zydena) is not FDA approved for sale in the United States, but is available in other countries.

Cialis is available in the following size tablets:

- 2.5 mg
- 5 mg
- 10 mg
- 20 mg

Viagra is available in the following size tablets:

- 25 mg
- 50 mg
- 100 mg

Levitra is available in the following size tablets:

- 2.5 mg
- 5 mg
- 10 mg
- 20 mg

Stendra is available in the following size tablets:

- 50 mg
- 100 mg
- 200 mg

The PDE5Is act by selectively preventing cyclic guanosine monophosphate (GMP) breakdown in the corpora cavernosa and the pulmonary arterial vasculature, which potentiates the downstream effects of nitric oxide. Nitric oxide induces smooth muscle relaxation and vasodilation through its effects on the cyclic GMP pathway. The molecular structure of sildenafil and the other PDE5Is is similar to cyclic GMP. This class of drug acts by binding competitively to PDE5, resulting in more cyclic GMP and increased duration of erections and pulmonary arterial vasodilation. The half-life of sildenafil, vardenafil, and avanfil is 3 to 5 hours, whereas the half-life of tadalafil is 17.5 hours. Sildenafil also weakly inhibits PDE6 with an efficacy of approximately one-tenth of that for PDE5. PDE6 is present in the photoreceptors in the retina and is an important component of the phototransduction cascade. Transient perception of blue after PDE5I use is due to binding to PDED6.

The primary indication for sildenafil is treatment of ED. Other uses include treatment of pulmonary arterial hypertension (approved by the FDA in 2005 as Revatio) and prevention and treatment of high-altitude pulmonary edema associated with altitude sickness. Tadalafil was approved by the FDA in 2009 for treatment of pulmonary arterial hypertension (Adcirca), and for treating benign prostatic hyperplasia in 2011. The recommended dosage of Revatio for pulmonary hypertension is 60 mg daily and therefore is close to the lowest dosage (50 mg) of Viagra. Adcirca is prescribed in a dosage of 40 mg daily for treatment of pulmonary arterial hypertension, which is greater than the highest dose of tadalafil used for treatment of ED.

Review of Case Reports of Association Between Phosphodiesterase-5 Inhibitors and Ischemic Optic Neuropathy

The first case of ischemic optic neuropathy associated with sildenafil use was reported in 2000 by Egan and Pomeranz,[1] followed by a second case reported by Cunningham and Smith[2] in 2001. These 2 cases were followed by case series reported in 2002 and 2005.[3,4] Numerous other single case reports or case series of ischemic optic neuropathy associated with sildenafil or tadalafil have since been published[5–24] (**Table 1**). There are 2 reported cases of combined retinal vascular occlusions and ischemic optic neuropathy.[15,16] As of 2015, 40 cases of ischemic optic neuropathy associated with PDE5I use have been reported in the peer-reviewed medical literature, including 3 cases in which PDE5I was used for treatment of pulmonary arterial hypertension[5,14,24] and 2 cases attributed to a Chinese herbal medicine containing sildenafil.[9,12] An optic neuropathy associated with the use of over-the-counter sexual enhancement supplements has been reported by Karli and colleagues,[25] but it is unclear whether or not this was an ischemic optic neuropathy because there was enhancement of the optic nerve on MRI. Three cases of posterior ischemic optic neuropathy associated with PDE5I have been reported, 2 of which occurred in children being treated for pulmonary arterial hypertension[5,14] and 1 in a 57-year-old man taking sildenafil for treatment of ED.[10] The FDA has also issued a warning on its Web site regarding variable amounts of PDE5I found in substances marketed for the purpose of enhancement of the sexual experience.

In addition to cases reported in the medical literature, the FDA has compiled cases of vision loss associated with PDE5I that have been reported to it through its Med-Watch Program. The details of vision loss are incomplete in most of these cases, because the reports can be provided by patients or other lay individuals in addition to physicians and pharmaceutical companies; therefore, they cannot be relied on to provide material for formal statistical analysis. However, they do provide an indirect indicator of the number of reported cases of NAION relative to the number of prescriptions dispensed for ED medications, as well as a sense of the magnitude of visual loss. According to the

Table 1
Characteristics of reported cases of NAION occurring after erectile dysfunction drug use

Reference	Age (mo)	Risk Factors	Notes	Final Acuity
Gaffuri et al,[5] 2014	7	CHD	Bilateral PION	Not known
Galvez-Ruiz & Arishi,[6] 2013	52	DM	100 mg sildenafil used at least 2–3 times/mo for 1 y	20/20, 20/40
	50	DM, IHD	Sildenafil routinely used for >1 y (dose not known)	20/300, 20/100
	52	DM	Sildenafil regularly used 2–3 times/wk for 2 y (dose not known)	20/25, 20/30
	41	DM	Sildenafil regularly used more than 2–3 times/wk (dose not known)	20/100, 20/30
	45	DM	Sildenafil regularly used more than 2–3 times/wk for 6 mo (dose not known)	20/80, 20/30
	38	DM, HLD	Simultaneous bilateral vision loss after starting daily sildenafil (dose not known)	Not known
	56	HTN, HC	Sildenafil regularly used more than 2–3 times/wk for 6–8 mo (dose not known)	HM, CF
	51	DM, HLD	Sildenafil intake in the days before vision loss OU (dose not known)	20/25, 20/40
	52	DM, HTN	Sildenafil regularly used >2–3 times/wk for more than 1 y (dose not known)	20/60, 20/50
	70	DM, HLD	Sildenafil regularly taken for >2–3 mo (dose not known)	1/200, 1/200
Tarantini et al,[7] 2012	60	DM	16 h after the 3rd of 3 daily doses of 50 mg sildenafil	20/50
Felekis et al,[8] 2011	51	HC	Bilateral NAION 12 h post Viagra use	20/25 OU
Moschos & Margetis,[9] 2011	55	None	8 mo post continued use of sildenafil 4–5 times per month (dose not known)	20/20 OU
Cullen & Chung,[10] 2010	57	HTN	Bilateral PION, Chinese health product taken daily for 2 wk	CF OD, HM OS
El-Domyati et al,[11] 2009	48	None	36 h post 25 mg, then 50 mg sildenafil	CF

(*continued on next page*)

Table 1
(continued)

Reference	Age (mo)	Risk Factors	Notes	Final Acuity
Su et al,[12] 2008	76	HTN, HLD, stroke	Chinese herbal product 3 capsules before onset of vision loss	HM OD, CF OS
Pepin & Pitha-Rowe,[13] 2008	63	None	3-step sequential decline in vision (dose not known)	20/40
Sivaswamy & Vanstavern,[14] 2007	6	Pulmonary hypertension	10 mg sildenafil 3 times a day × 15 mo	LP
Gedik et al,[15] 2007	36	Chronic renal failure	The next morning after ingestion of 100 mg sildenafil for each eye	20/25 OU
Akash et al,[16] 2005	54	None	NAION and CAO a few hours after ingestion of 200 mg sildenafil	HM
Gruhn & Fledelius,[17] 2005	69	None	18 h after ingestion of 50 mg sildenafil	20/20
Dheer et al,[18] 2002	48	None	After ingestion of 100 mg sildenafil daily × 2 d	20/20
Pomeranz & Bhavsar,[4] 2005	59	None	A few hours after ingestion of 25 mg sildenafil	LP OD, HM OS
	58	HC	1 h after ingestion after 50 mg sildenafil	HM
	67	HTN	Next day after ingestion of 50 mg sildenafil	20/200
	69	HTN	24 h after ingestion of 100 mg sildenafil	20/125
	50	None	30 h after ingestion of 100 mg sildenafil	20/160
	66	HTN, HLD, DM	36 h after ingestion (dose not known)	20/25
	60	HTN, HLD	Next morning after ingestion (dose not known)	20/20
Pomeranz et al,[3] 2002	52	Prostate cancer, Crohn	60 min after ingestion of 50 mg sildenafil	20/20
	69	HC	45 min after ingestion of sildenafil	20/80
	42	None	12 h after ingestion of sildenafil (dose not known)	20/200
	62	NAION OS	50 mg sildenafil weekly for 15 mo	20/50
	59	DM, smoking, CAD	Several hours after ingestion of 50 mg sildenafil	20/25
Peter et al,[19] 2005	59	None	7 d post 20 mg tadalafil	20/30
Escaravage et al,[20] 2005	59	None	45 h post 20 mg tadalafil	20/20

(*continued on next page*)

Table 1
(*continued*)

Reference	Age (mo)	Risk Factors	Notes	Final Acuity
Bollinger & Lee,[21] 2005	67	HC	5 episodes of challenge/ rechallenge with 20 mg tadalafil	20/30
Kim & Kim,[22] 2012	54	Smoking	100 mg udenafil ingested 12 h before vision loss	20/20
Prat et al,[24] 2011	63	Pulmonary hypertension, chronic vascular disease	50 mg sildenafil 3 times a day, bilateral NAION 1 mo apart	HM, CF

Abbreviations: CAD, coronary artery disease; CAO, cilioretinal artery occlusion; CF, counting fingers; CHD, congenital heart disease; DM, diabetes; HC, hypercholesterolemia; HLD, hyperlipidemia; HM, hand motions; HTN, hypertension; IHD, ischemic heart disease; NAION, nonarteritic anterior ischemic optic neuropathy; OU, both eyes; PION, posterior ischemic optic neuropathy.

Adapted from Pomeranz HD. The relationship between phosphodiesterase-5 inhibitors and nonarteritic anterior ischemic optic neuropathy. J Neuroophthalmol 2016;36(2):193–6; with permission.

FDA's Web site, 43 cases of ischemic optic neuropathy associated with PDE5I use had been reported to the FDA Adverse Event Reporting System (AERS) as of 2005. Pomeranz[26] analyzed the data in the AERS as of December 2014 and found that the FDA had received reports of 553 cases of ischemic optic neuropathy associated with PDE5I use. This is significantly higher than the number of cases reported in the peer-reviewed medical literature and may possibly more accurately reflect how frequently ischemic optic neuropathy occurs in individuals prescribed PDE5I.

Research Studies Investigating Effects of Phosphodiesterase-5 Inhibitors on Ocular Circulation

The effects of sildenafil on the arterial blood supply to the eye have been studied in healthy volunteers as well as on individuals with known ED.

- Grunwald and colleagues[27] studied the effect of 100 mg sildenafil in 15 healthy volunteers with laser Doppler flowmetry and concluded that sildenafil caused no significant change in optic nerve rim or foveolar choroidal blood flow, and no effect on retinal vascular caliber.[28]
- Kurtulan and colleagues[29] reported that 100 mg sildenafil had no effect on ocular hemodynamics of the central retinal artery on the basis of color Doppler ultrasonography in 38 patients with ED.
- In an investigation of 20 subjects with ED given 100 mg sildenafil, Koksal and colleagues[30] reported that peak systolic velocity, end-diastolic velocity, and mean velocity were significantly increased 1 hour after drug intake in the ophthalmic and short posterior ciliary arteries, but not the central retinal artery.
- Dündar and colleagues[31] found no changes in color Doppler hemodynamics in the ophthalmic, central retinal, and short posterior ciliary arteries in 15 patients with ED who received 50 mg sildenafil twice a week for 3 months.
- An increase in pulsatile ocular blood flow caused by a change in the choroidal vasculature was reported by Paris and colleagues[32] in 12 healthy adults after ingestion of a 50-mg dose of sildenafil.

- Pache and colleagues[33] reported a significant dilatation of retinal arteries and veins in healthy subjects after 50 mg sildenafil using a retinal vessel analyzer.
- Polak and colleagues[34] reported that sildenafil increases retinal venous diameters and retinal blood flow in healthy volunteers after 100 mg sildenafil using laser Doppler flowmetry and retinal vessel analyzer.
- McCulley and colleagues[35] found that 200 mg sildenafil caused small inconsistent changes in choroidal thickness in healthy volunteers.
- Vance and colleagues[36] studied the effects of 100 mg sildenafil on choroidal thickness in 4 healthy men and 4 healthy women using enhanced-depth optic coherence tomography and found that choroidal thickness increased by 12% at 1 and 3 hours after ingestion compared with baseline.
- Kim and colleagues[37] measured choroidal perfusion and thickness in 7 healthy male subjects following ingestion of 50 mg sildenafil at 2 hours and confirmed increased choroidal perfusion and thickness.

An animal model for ischemic optic neuropathy has been established in rodents and primates and has been used to study the mechanism by which damage occurs to the optic nerve after circulation has been disrupted.[38–42] These models use laser light to activate an intravascular photoactive dye to induce capillary vascular thrombosis and result in changes to the optic nerve that are indistinguishable from that seen in clinical disease. It does not appear that any studies have been published using the animal model for NAION to determine whether or not administration of PDE5I affects damage to the optic nerve.

The previously described studies show that

- Sildenafil has minimal effect on the retinal, optic disk, and choroidal arterial circulation in healthy individuals.
- The effect of sildenafil in study participants with ED was variable depending on the study.
- No studies were specifically directed at individuals with significant risk factors for NAION, such as a history of nocturnal hypotension, sleep apnea, or NAION in the fellow eye or a small cup-to-disk ratio.
- Animal models of ischemic optic neuropathy have not as yet been used to assess whether PDE5I administration affects the extent of damage to the optic nerve.

Epidemiologic Investigations Regarding Phosphodiesterase-5 Inhibitor Use and Nonarteritic Anterior Ischemic Optic Neuropathy

A case-control study of PDE5I and NAION was found to be feasible using a National Veterans Health Administration's pharmacy and clinical databases.[43] McGwin and colleagues[44] conducted a retrospective case-control study with 38 cases of NAION and 389 controls who participated in a telephone interview regarding past and current use of Viagra and Cialis, but the interviewers were not blinded to case status. They found a statistically significant association between ED drug use and NAION in those subjects with a history of myocardial infarction. Sobel and Cappelleri from Pfizer[45] criticized the conclusions of McGwin and colleagues[44] based on methodological limitations, such as study biases, sample size, and statistical analysis, ultimately resulting in a retraction of the study by McGwin and colleagues[44] in 2011.

A nested case-control study[46] of a health claims database using physician diagnostic codes and prescription medication dispensed identified cases of NAION that were matched with corresponding controls and correlated with the prescription of PDE5I. A conditional logistic regression model was used to estimate the likelihood of an association between NAION and the prescription of PDE5I. The investigators concluded that there was no association between PDE5I prescription and NAION. The design of study was limited solely to diagnostic codes and prescriptions identified in a database. No "real" data (ie, patient cases of NAION or direct linkage of patients to an actual prescription record of PDE5I use) were used in this study. Other weaknesses of this study were the assumptions that writing a prescription for a PDE5I always resulted in it being ingested by the patient, the patient did not receive prescriptions from other sources, and patients did not obtain PDE5I through another source.

Prospective Studies of Nonarteritic Anterior Ischemic Optic Neuropathy and Phosphodiesterase-5 Inhibitor Use Mandated by the Food and Drug Administration

In 2005, after extensive publicity regarding a possible association between PDE5I use and NAION, the FDA mandated that Pfizer, Bayer, and Eli Lilly place warnings on their drug inserts and perform prospective observational studies to determine whether or not there was an association between PDE5I and NAION. Pfizer's study results were reported in August 2013 on the National Institutes of Health clinical trials Web site and have been published elsewhere.[47] Studies by Bayer and Eli Lilly are still ongoing (see clinicaltrials.org).

Pfizer carried out a case-crossover retrospective study. The primary outcome measure was the number of cases of definite NAION that had been exposed to a PDE5I during a 1-day case window (ie, the day before symptomatic onset of vision loss) compared with the rest of the 30-day period before vision loss. A case was considered "associated" if sildenafil or vardenafil was used on that day and/or the previous day, or if tadalafil was used that day and/or any of the previous 4 days because of its longer half-life. Seventy-six potential NAION cases with PDE5I exposure were identified. Of these, 43 cases were deemed to be definite NAION and 21 to be possible NAION. Of these 43 definite NAION cases, 14 cases were exposed to PDE5I during the day before symptom onset. Based on conditional logistic regression, an odds ratio of 2.15 was calculated for developing definite NAION the day after exposure to PDE5I, and for combined definite and possible cases of NAION, increased to 2.36.

The results strongly suggest an increased risk of developing NAION after ingestion of a PDE5I. The major limitation of this study was that it relied on retrospective recall of PDE5I use. The main strength of this study was the case-crossover design that controlled for personal characteristics over the study period. In response to the results of this prospective research study by Pfizer, the FDA mandated an update to the drug warning for the PDE5I in March 2014.

SUMMARY

- Forty cases of ischemic optic neuropathy associated with PDE5I have been documented in peer-reviewed publications, the details of which vary significantly in terms of
  - The frequency with which these drugs were ingested before onset of vision loss
  - The dose of drug consumed
  - The time interval between last use of drug and onset of vision loss
- Many, though not all, cases had microvascular risk factors associated with ischemic optic neuropathy.
- There have not been any reported investigations of the effect of PDE5I on ocular circulation in individuals with microvascular disease and/or the "disk at risk," so it is not known whether such individuals carry a higher risk for development of NAION in association with ingestion of PDE5I.

- There are no convincing epidemiologic studies linking NAION with PDE5I.
- However, Pfizer's case-crossover study documented a twofold increase in risk of NAION in individuals who ingested sildenafil or tadalafil within the previous 24 hours.

The following is recommended regarding NAION and PDE5I use:

- If NAION occurs, an inquiry should be made as to whether any PDE5I medication has been used for
  - Treatment of ED (in men)
  - Pulmonary arterial hypertension (men and women or children)
  - Whether the patient has used any substance marketed for the purpose of enhancement of sexual experience, many of which have been determined by the FDA to include variable amounts of PDE5I medications among their ingredients
- If so, the patient should be counseled as to
  - The future likelihood of development of NAION in the fellow eye, which is recognized from the Ischemic Optic Neuropathy Decompression Trial to be approximately 15%.
  - The possibility that continued PDE5I use may additionally increase the risk of NAION. As noted previously, the Pfizer observational study demonstrated at least a twofold increased risk. Whether or not this makes the overall potential risk of fellow eye involvement with continued PDE5I use as high as 30% has yet to be determined.
- Patients with a previous known history of occurrence of NAION in one eye should be discouraged from use of PDE5I for treatment of ED or pulmonary arterial hypertension because of the increased risk of fellow eye involvement.

REFERENCES

1. Egan R, Pomeranz H. Sildenafil (Viagra) associated anterior ischemic optic neuropathy. Arch Ophthalmol 2000;118:291–2.
2. Cunningham AV, Smith KH. Anterior ischemic optic neuropathy associated with Viagra. J Neuroophthalmol 2001;21:22–5.
3. Pomeranz HD, Smith KH, Hart WM Jr, et al. Sildenafil-associated nonarteritic anterior ischemic optic neuropathy. Ophthalmology 2002;109:584–7.
4. Pomeranz HD, Bhavsar AR. Non-arteritic ischemic optic neuropathy developing soon after use of sildenafil (Viagra): a report of seven new cases. J Neuroophthalmol 2005;25:9–13.
5. Gaffuri M, Cristofaletti A, Mansoldo C, et al. Acute onset of bilateral visual loss during sildenafil therapy in a young infant with congenital heart disease. BMJ Case Rep 2014;2014.
6. Galvez-Ruiz A, Arishi N. Sequential, non-arteritic anterior ischemic optic neuropathy in patients taking sildenafil: a report of ten cases. Saudi J Ophthalmol 2013;27:241–6.
7. Tarantini A, Faraoni A, Menchini F, et al. Bilateral simultaneous non-arteritic anterior ischemic optic neuropathy after ingestion of sildenafil for erectile dysfunction. Case Rep Med 2012;747:658.
8. Felekis T, Asproudis I, Katsanos K, et al. A case of non-arteritic anterior ischemic optic neuropathy of a male with family history of the disease after receiving sildenafil. Clin Ophthalmol 2011;5:1443–5.
9. Moschos MM, Margetis I. Bilateral simultaneous anterior ischemic optic neuropathy associated with sildenafil. Case Rep Ophthalmol 2011;2:262–5.

10. Cullen JF, Chung HW. Mistaken diagnosis of optic neuritis and the possible role of phosphodiesterase-5 inhibitors (Sildenafil/Viagra). Med J Malaysia 2010;65: 315–6.
11. El-Domyati MM, El-Fakahany HM, Morad KE. Non-arteritic ischaemic optic neuropathy (NAION) after 36 h of intake of sildenafil citrate: first Egyptian case. Andrologia 2009;41:319–21.
12. Su DH, Ang PS, Tow SL. Bilateral posterior ischemic optic neuropathy associated with use of sildenafil. J Neuroophthalmol 2008;28:75.
13. Pepin S, Pitha-Rowe I. Stepwise decline in visual field after serial sildenafil use. J Neuroophthalmol 2008;28:76–7.
14. Sivaswamy L, Vanstavern GP. Ischemic optic neuropathy in a child. Pediatr Neurol 2007;37:371–2.
15. Gedik S, Yilmaz G, Akova YA. Sildenafil-associated consecutive non-arteritic anterior ischaemic optic neuropathy, cilioretinal artery occlusion, and central retinal vein occlusion in a haemodialysis patient. Eye (Lond) 2007;21:129–30.
16. Akash R, Hrishikesh D, Amith P, et al. Case report: association of combined non-arteritic anterior ischemic optic neuropathy (NAION) and obstruction of cilioretinal artery with overdose of Viagra. J Ocul Pharmacol Ther 2005;21:315–7.
17. Gruhn N, Fledelius HC. Unilateral optic neuropathy associated with sildenafil intake. Acta Ophthalmol Scand 2005;83:131–2.
18. Dheer S, Rekhi GS, Merlyn S. Sildenafil associated anterior ischaemic optic neuropathy. J Assoc Physicians India 2002;50:265.
19. Peter NM, Singh MV, Fox PD. Tadalafil-associated anterior ischaemic optic neuropathy. Eye (Lond) 2005;19:715–7.
20. Escaravage GK Jr, Wright JD Jr, Givre SJ. Tadalafil associated with anterior ischemic optic neuropathy. Arch Ophthalmol 2005;123:399–400.
21. Bollinger K, Lee MS. Recurrent visual field defect and ischemic optic neuropathy associated with tadalafil rechallenge. Arch Ophthalmol 2005;123:400–1.
22. Kim IG, Kim DY. Anterior ischemic optic neuropathy associated with udenafil. Korean J Ophthalmol 2012;26:235–8.
23. Hafidi Z, Handor H, Laghmari M, et al. Cilioretinal artery and central retinal vein occlusion after sildenafil use. Emerg Med J 2014;31:535.
24. Prat NM, Sanchez-Dalmau BF, Foroozan R. Not just for men. Surv Ophthalmol 2011;56:173–7.
25. Karli SZ, Liao SD, Carey AR, et al. Optic neuropathy associated with use of over-the-counter sexual enhancement supplements. Clin Ophthalmol 2014;8:2171–5.
26. Pomeranz HD. Cases of ischemic optic neuropathy associated with phosphodiesterase-5 inhibitor use reported to the Food and Drug Administration Adverse Event Reporting System. J Neuroophthalmol 2016;36(2):221–2.
27. Grunwald JE, Siu KK, Jacob SS, et al. Effect of sildenafil citrate (Viagra) on the ocular circulation. Am J Ophthalmol 2001;131:751–5.
28. Grunwald JE, Metelitsina T, Grunwald L. Effect of sildenafil citrate (Viagra) on retinal blood vessel diameter. Am J Ophthalmol 2002;133:809–12.
29. Kurtulan E, Gulcu A, Secil M, et al. Effects of sildenafil on ocular perfusion demonstrated by color Doppler ultrasonography. Int J Impot Res 2004;16:244–8.
30. Koksal M, Ozdemir H, Kargi S, et al. The effects of sildenafil on ocular blood flow. Acta Ophthalmol Scand 2005;83:355–9.
31. Dündar SO, Dayanir Y, Topaloğlu A, et al. Effect of sildenafil on ocular hemodynamics in 3 months regular use. Int J Impot Res 2006;18:282–6.
32. Paris G, Sponsel WE, Sandoval SS, et al. Sildenafil increases ocular perfusion. Int Ophthalmol 2001;23:355–8.

33. Pache M, Meyer P, Prünte C, et al. Sildenafil induces retinal vasodilatation in healthy subjects. Br J Ophthalmol 2002;86:156–8.
34. Polak K, Wimpissinger B, Berisha F, et al. Effects of sildenafil on retinal blood flow and flicker-induced retinal vasodilatation in healthy subjects. Invest Ophthalmol Vis Sci 2003;44:4872–6.
35. McCulley TJ, Luu JK, Marmor MF, et al. Effects of sildenafil citrate (Viagra) on choroidal congestion. Ophthalmologica 2002;216:455–8.
36. Vance SK, Imamura Y, Freund KB. The effects of sildenafil citrate on choroidal thickness as determined by enhance depth imaging optical coherence tomography. Retina 2011;31:332–5.
37. Kim OY, Silverman RH, Chan KV, et al. Measurement of choroidal perfusion and thickness following system sildenafil (Viagra). Acta Ophthalmol 2013;91:183–8.
38. Wang Y, Brown DP, Watson BD, et al. Rat model of photochemically-induced posterior ischemic optic neuropathy. J Vis Exp 2015;105:e52402.
39. Bernstein SL, Miller NR. Ischemic optic neuropathies and their models: disease comparisons, model strengths and weaknesses. Jpn J Ophthalmol 2015;59: 135–47.
40. Bernstein SL, Johnson MA, Miller NR. Nonarteritic anterior ischemic optic neuropathy (NAION) and its experimental models. Prog Retin Eye Res 2011;30:167–87.
41. Bernstein SL, Guo Y, Kelman SE, et al. Functional and cellular responses in a novel rodent model of anterior ischemic optic neuropathy. Invest Ophthalmol Vis Sci 2003;44:4153–62.
42. Chen CS, Johnson MA, Flower RA, et al. A primate model of nonarteritic anterior ischemic optic neuropathy. Invest Ophthalmol Vis Sci 2008;49:2985–92.
43. Margo CE, French DD. Ischemic optic neuropathy in male veterans prescribed phosphodiesterase-5 inhibitors. Am J Ophthalmol 2007;143:538–9.
44. McGwin G Jr, Vaphiades MS, Hall TA, et al. Non-arteritic anterior ischaemic optic neuropathy and the treatment of erectile dysfunction. Br J Ophthalmol 2006;90: 154–7.
45. Sobel RE, Cappelleri JC. NAION and treatment of erectile dysfunction: reply from Pfizer. Br J Ophthalmol 2006;90:927.
46. Nathoo NA, Etminan M, Mikelberg FS. Association between phosphodiesterase 5 inhibitors and non-arteritic anterior ischemic optic neuropathy. J Neuroophthalmol 2015;35:12–5.
47. Campbell NB, Walker AM, Gaffney M, et al. Acute nonarteritic anterior ischemic optic neuropathy and exposure to phosphodiesterase type 5 inhibitors. J Sex Med 2015;12:139–51.

Homonymous Hemianopia and Vision Restoration Therapy

Alexander Frolov, MD[a], Jeanne Feuerstein, MD[a],
Prem S. Subramanian, MD, PhD[b,*]

KEYWORDS

• Vision restoration therapy • Homonymous hemianopia • Stroke • Visual field loss
• Visual rehabilitation • CNS plasticity

KEY POINTS

- Acquired hemianopia is disabling and there is currently no standardized rehabilitation for patients with this deficit.
- Compensatory techniques and devices aimed at improving function are common, but are not validated in large randomized controlled trials.
- Plasticity in the visual pathway may allow for repair of visual field loss that was previously assumed to be static.
- Visual restoration therapy is a rehabilitation method that purports to enlarge the visual field in patients with hemianopia, but remains a controversial topic.

INTRODUCTION

Although the debilitating motor and language effects of stroke and other brain injury are well-known and systematically addressed as part of early and intensive rehabilitation efforts,[1] visual disturbance is less often described and is only secondarily targeted during rehabilitation, if at all. Among patients with acquired hemianopia secondary to stroke, the nature of the deficit can vary widely, depending on the location of the lesion and the part of the visual pathway that is disrupted, and recovery and functional improvement are adversely affected even when severity of stroke and motor deficits are controlled for.[2,3] Despite this, rehabilitation strategies for visual loss are neither standardized nor ubiquitous. This remains the case for varied reasons, the foremost

Disclosure Statement: The authors have nothing to disclose.
[a] Department of Neurology, University of Colorado School of Medicine, Aurora, CO 80045, USA; [b] Department of Ophthalmology, University of Colorado School of Medicine, Mail Stop F731, 1675 Aurora Court, Aurora, CO 80045, USA
* Corresponding author.
E-mail address: prem.subramanian@ucdenver.edu

Neurol Clin 35 (2017) 29–43
http://dx.doi.org/10.1016/j.ncl.2016.08.010

being that visual deficits after injury are generally considered to be permanent and not amenable to rehabilitation.[3]

In the last 2 decades, techniques focused on improving visual deficits have emerged alongside an established body of visual aids and training regimens aimed to overcome a fixed visual deficit. These established strategies and aids have their benefits and drawbacks, but none of them directly use neuroplasticity as a means to regain lost vision. New data, on the other hand, suggests that there is significant plasticity in the adult visual pathway, which may affect actual improvement in the damaged visual field.[4–8] With these data in mind, a computer-based training system termed visual restoration therapy (VRT) and commercialized under the moniker NovaVision (NovaVision, Inc, Bowling Green, OH) was created in the late 1990s.[9] Although initial studies examining VRT showed promise in decreasing the size of the scotoma and improving patients' subjective visual experience, subsequent controversy regarding outcome measures, perimetry data, and cost to clinical benefit ratio arose. This review presents strategies in use for visual restoration and adaptation, the data for and against VRT, visual system plasticity research, and the arguments surrounding the evidence available.

SCOPE OF THE PROBLEM

The human visual system is a complex and crossed system consisting of several connections and projections, organized in a topographic manner from the retina to the primary visual cortex in the occipital lobe. After light enters the eye and strikes the rods and cones of the retina, this information travels to the ganglion cells of the retina, and then projects to the brain via the optic nerve. Axons receiving input from the temporal visual field (and thus the nasal retina) cross at the optic chasm joining the contralateral optic tract, while the axons with nasal visual field input (and thus the temporal retina) form part of the ipsilateral optic tract. While the axons in the optic tract travel to multiple regions of the brain, the vast majority project to the lateral geniculate nucleus of the thalamus. From the thalamus, they project to the primary visual cortex in the occipital lobe via the optic radiations. Information continues upstream from the primary visual cortex to various secondary processing areas involved in language tasks, spatial orientation, color perception, and other complex functions.

Localizing clinical deficits along the retinogeniculostriate pathway is fairly straightforward. When an injury is retrochiasmal, a homonymous visual field defect is usually found. For example, an injury to the left optic tract immediately posterior to the optic chiasm causes a right homonymous hemianopia, as will injury to the left occipital lobe (although the density of the deficit may vary). The exact type of homonymous defect (complete hemianopia, quadrantanopia, scotoma, etc) depends largely on the exact location of the injury, the extent of the injury, and the presence of other injuries (**Fig. 1**).

Completed ischemic infarcts are not expected to worsen after initial injury, unless new injury occurs. Poststroke treatment thus includes identification of the stroke etiology, risk factor modification to prevent recurrences, and initiation of early and intensive rehabilitation to optimize functional outcomes. Such intensive rehabilitation has been shown to improve disability and independence after stroke, and even to reduce mortality.[1,2,10–12] In most hospitals rehabilitation targets motor, language, and cognitive dysfunction, using physical, occupational, and speech therapy teams to evaluate and treat the patient from day 1 of injury. In contrast, there is no standardized treatment for visual deficits in the acute period after a stroke, and few data exist on this topic.[3,13] As a result, patients with homonymous visual deficits are often taught compensatory strategies in the acute and subacute settings, and treatments that

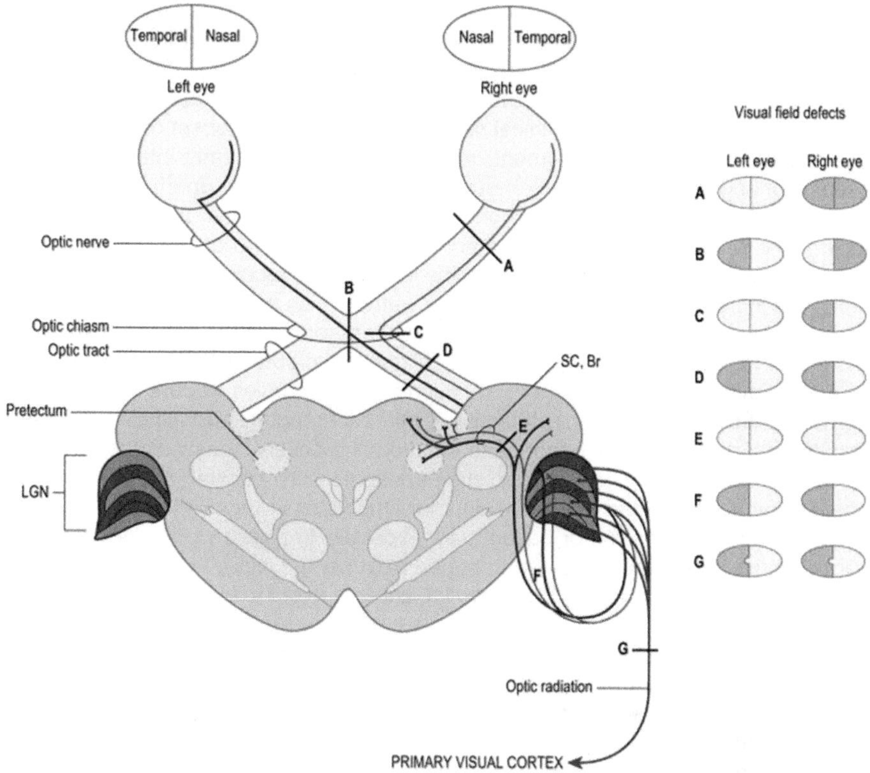

Fig. 1. Visual field defects associated with lesions of the visual pathway. The bars (*A–G*) depict the location of lesions, and the associated visual field defect is shown at the right (shaded area represents visual field loss). *A*: Lesion of the right optic nerve causes blindness in the right eye. *B*: Optic chiasm lesion results in a bitemporal hemianopia, a loss of vision in the temporal visual field of both eyes. *C*: Lesion affecting only the uncrossed fibers of the optic chiasm results in a loss of vision in the nasal field of the ipsilateral eye. *D*: Lesion of the optic tract causes homonymous hemianopia, or complete loss of vision in the contralateral visual field. An afferent pupillary defect also arises from a lesion at this level. *E*: Lesion affecting the fibers in the brachium of the superior colliculus (SC, Br) results in an afferent pupillary defect, but with intact visual fields because the projection to the lateral geniculate nucleus (LGN) remains intact. *F*: Lesions at the level of the LGN are similar to lesions at D and result in homonymous hemianopia, but with an intact, normal pupillary reflex. *G*: Lesions at the level of the optic radiation also result in a homonymous hemianopia, but with sparing of macular vision. (*From* Matsubara JA, Boyd JD. Overview of the central visual pathways. In: Levin LA, Nilsson SFE, Ver Hoeve J, et al. Adler's physiology of the eye. 11th edition. Philadelphia: Saunders Elsevier, 2011; with permission.)

target visual deficit are implemented years to months after injury, if at all. These include continued practice of compensatory strategies, as well as the use of optical aids, without focus on improving the visual field.[14] However, research shows that homonymous visual deficits worsen functional outcomes and independence levels, even when severity of concurrent motor deficits is controlled for.[1–3]

Spontaneous recovery of visual field deficits after injury is common and well-demonstrated.[3,4,8,14–16] This recovery is variable, and is likely related to the degree of neuronal death and stunning in the damaged visual pathways, as well as to resolution of the initial effects of acute injury (ie, inflammation and edema). PET studies demonstrate recovery of metabolic activity in the striate cortex in patients with resolving homonymous visual field deficits; in contrast, there is no such metabolic recovery in those with persistent clinical deficits.[3] Identifying the subset of patients who will show spontaneous improvement, and studying whether early intervention can speed up or augment this recovery, has proven difficult, however. Spontaneous recovery is expected early, and after 2 months is likely complete.[14–16] In a retrospective study, 40% of 263 patients with homonymous hemianopia of various etiologies showed spontaneous improvement, and the likelihood of recovery decreased significantly with increased time from injury.[16] (The authors also note that the 40% figure is falsely low because many of the patients likely had spontaneous improvement even before their first formal visual evaluation, highlighting the potential difficulties in studying interventions in this patient population.) Other studies report spontaneous improvement in 50% to 60% of patients within the first month, and almost none after 3 months.[13] Additionally, the degree and duration of recovery is likely impacted by the type and severity of injury (ie, ischemic stroke patients with occipital lobe injury are expected to regain use of the ischemic penumbra that is reperfused in the first few days after the insult, whereas tumor patients are expected to regain vision depending on change in tumor or edema size after targeted treatment). Finally, the data on spontaneous recovery remains largely retrospective and is subject to the inherent limitations of such analyses (**Fig. 2**).

Visual field recovery has been postulated to occur from both improved function of injured tissue and recruitment of additional cortical structures to assume the function of the permanently damaged centers.[4,8,13] A number of studies demonstrate plasticity in the mammalian visual system that is distinct from early spontaneous recovery.[5–7,17,18] This plasticity may underlie behavioral compensatory strategies, improvement in visual tasks after training, and less understood clinical entities such as blindsight.[a] Huxlin's research performed in cats[5,6] demonstrates that damage to extrastriate areas (such as the lateral suprasylvian cortex) creates deficits in the ability to integrate motion signals and extract motion signals from noise. One study[6] used an intensive retraining protocol in the impaired hemifield, teaching the animals to discriminate motion direction. These animals demonstrated gradual recovery in motion integration after 15 to 40 days of intensive training. Moreover, this improvement remained stable over the next several months. In addition, evaluation of the neurochemical patterns in neurons subserving these extrastriate pathways showed changes in excitatory neuronal function and expression of excitatory receptor subunits after visual retraining, suggesting that plasticity in neuronal interconnections is driven by this training.[5] Similar data show improvement after retraining of monkeys with both striate[19,20] and extrastriate lesions.[21,22] For example, training of monkeys with striate lesions to make saccades into their blind hemifield and detect points of light led to improvements in the ability to detect stimuli within the blind visual field.[13]

In humans, significant controversy exists regarding the extent of plasticity and ability for recovery in the visual system. As early as 1917, research groups developed training

---

[a] Blindsight refers to the often unconscious existence of residual visual perception of things such as motion and form after V1 damage, seen in both human and animal studies. Although reviewing the mechanisms subserving blindsight is beyond the scope of this work, the basic principle of blindsight is the existence of visual pathways that entirely bypass V1, transmitting information from the retina and/or the lateral geniculate nucleus of the thalamus to extrastriate areas such as V4, V2, superior colliculus, and others.[8]

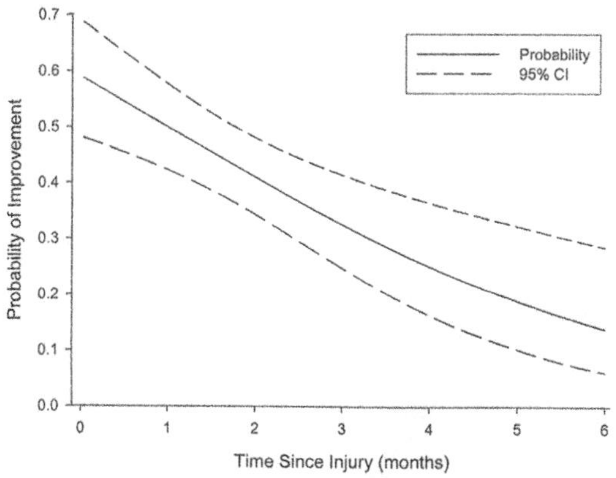

Fig. 2. Recovery from homonymous hemianopic defects in a cohort of 218 patients evaluated within 6 months of the injury causing the visual field loss, with probability of recovery plotted against time since injury. (*Reprinted from* Zhang X, Kedar S, Lynn MJ, et al. Natural history of homonymous hemianopia. Neurology 2006;66:901–5; with permission.)

protocols for patients with homonymous visual defects, and reported improvements in both functional status and actual visual field size.[23–25] The latter claim is especially controversial, however, because the perimetric methods used to evaluate the size of the scotoma (and thus to document reductions in its size) likely did not control for small shifts in fixation and quick saccades into the blind hemifield.[5,13,26] Despite this limitation, there is evidence of cortical reorganization after insult to the human visual system. Dilks and colleagues[7] described a patient who suffered a stroke which preserved the primary visual cortex (V1) but destroyed fibers from the upper left visual field, leading to a left upper quadrantanopia. The patient's perception in his left lower visual field became distorted, such that objects seemed elongated and stretched into the (blind) left upper visual field. Behavioral testing and functional MRI data in this patient revealed V1 reorganization (activation of the deprived V1 region with stimulation in the left lower visual field), demonstrating cortical plasticity in the visual system. In addition, Huxlin and colleagues[18] demonstrated that global discrimination training in 7 adults with V1 damage after stroke improved direction integration in the blind hemifield, with eye movements controlled for. Significantly, this improvement was retinotopically specific, meaning that the perceptual improvement was isolated to only the areas of the blind hemifield that were trained, and other areas of the blind hemifield revealed no improvement in perception. These patients also reported conscious awareness of improvement in their blind hemifield (**Fig. 3**).

COMPENSATORY STRATEGIES FOR HOMONYMOUS VISUAL DEFECTS

Although no standardized rehabilitation exists for homonymous visual defects, both devices and compensatory strategies have long been used to help these patients improve their functional status.[3,4,14,27] None of these strategies aim to enlarge the patient's true visual field. Instead, they focus on either relocating the blind hemifield into the patient's line of sight or honing voluntary compensatory eye and head movements to scan the blind hemifield more effectively.

Visual scanning in patients with homonymous hemianopias is disorganized and inaccurate, with prolonged and imprecise saccades leading to longer search and

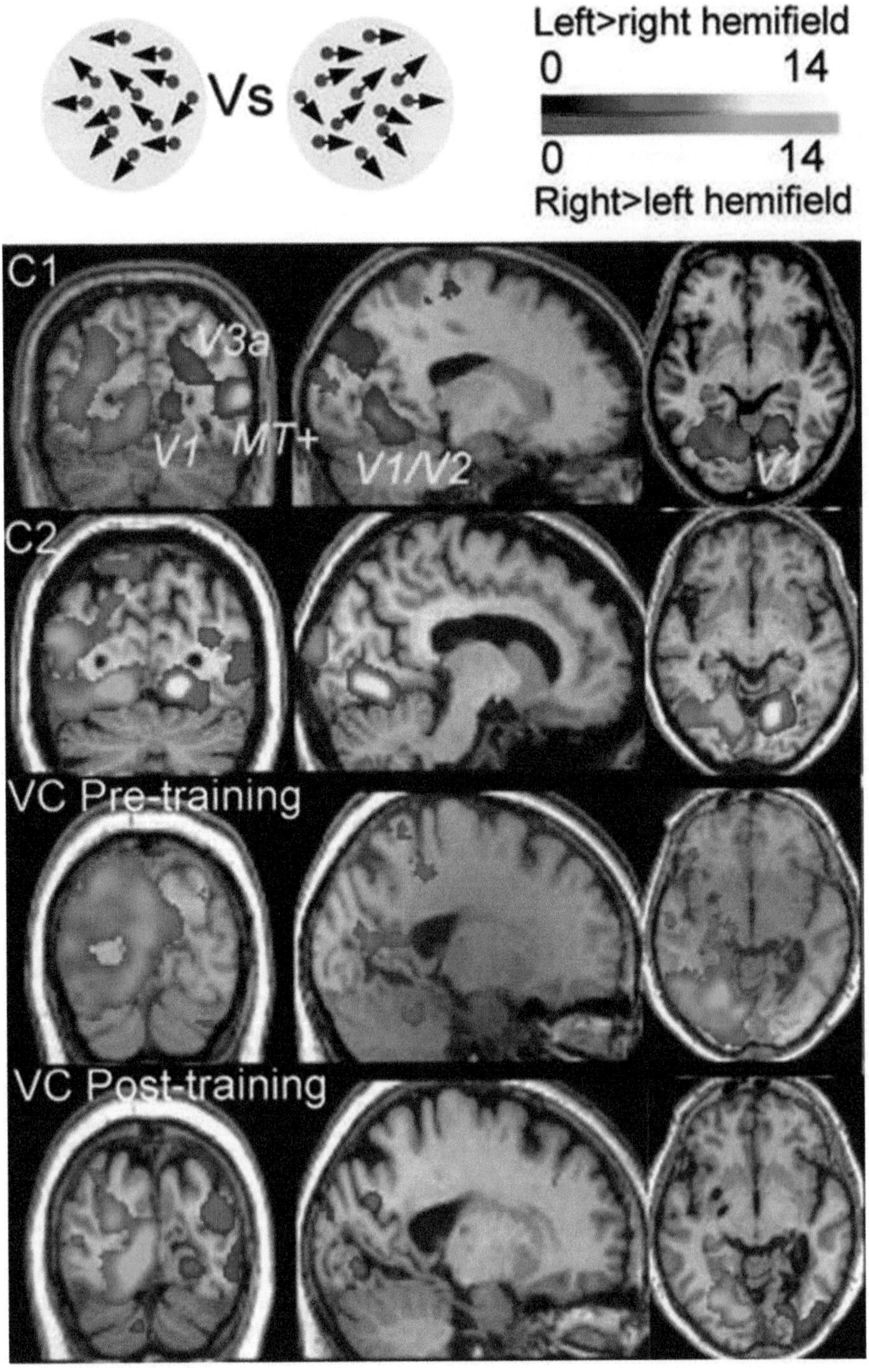

Fig. 3. Functional MRI data on normal control subjects (C1, C2) and a subject with visual cortex damage (VC) when asked to perform a global direction discrimination task. The VC patient shows hyperexcitation of the undamaged hemisphere and no activity in the lesioned side before training; afterward, there a more normal pattern of excitation in the normal

fixation times.[3,8] Research shows that for the 6 months after injury, eye movements and fixation patterns are similar to controls, whereas after 6 months these patterns are altered significantly.[3] For example, patients with hemianopia tend to look toward their blind hemifield, even when confronted with visual scanning tasks. In addition, patients searching for targets in their blind hemifield perform a series of hypometric saccades that approach the target until it is found. After the target is found, the saccades become hypermetric with a subsequent corrective saccade back to the target.[13] These natural compensatory strategies have been adapted into formal training protocols, which teach the patient how to consciously plan appropriate saccades and scanning strategies to more effectively bring the blind hemifield into the intact one in an organized and systematic fashion. These training strategies have been shown to improve the search fields of hemianopic patients by 10°, reduce the time to find objects by up to 50%, and improve patients' sense of impairment.[3,28,29] Unfortunately, large, randomized controlled trials (RCTs) for this intervention do not exist, and no data exist to guide optimal timing or frequency of such training.

Optical aids work by either relocating the visual information received by the hemianopic field onto the normal visual field, or by expanding the normal visual field.[3,27] Fresnel prisms (plastic press-on lenses that are fitted onto standard glasses) can be either monocular or binocular. Binocular application on the hemianopic side of the visual field helps to relocate the image into the normal part of the visual field, but does so only when gaze is focused into the prism, and thus does not provide true visual field expansion. Monocular application, of which there is more than 1 method, also improves the visual field when gaze is directed into the prism.[3] A small RCT of monocular prism application demonstrated improvement in visual tasks but not in activities of daily living, raising the question of the clinical significance of this method.[30] Another small, noncontrolled study evaluated monocular prism application with patients demonstrating a 20° visual field expansion by standard perimetry and functional improvement by report.[31] Use of obliquely oriented high-power sector Fresnel prisms (**Fig. 4**) has been commercialized, but many patients find the prisms disorienting and fail to adapt to their use. Although visual aids may help some patients and improve the visual field to a degree, the overall clinical usefulness is unknown owing to a lack of large RCTs.

VISUAL RESTORATION THERAPY

In the 1990s, a group headed by Bernhard Sabel and Erich Kasten published promising data regarding the effectiveness of a computer-based system for VRT, subsequently commercialized under the name NovaVision.[9] The system targets the border zone between the intact visual field and the scotoma with suprathreshold light stimuli. The stimulus is postulated to recruit residual intact neurons in border zone areas between the intact visual field and the scotoma, stimulating any inherent plasticity in the visual system and thereby increasing the size of the visual field and reducing the size of the scotoma. Using animal data showing restoration of visual function after damage[32,33] as scientific justification for their approach, Sabel and Kasten[9] described the results of 2 small clinical trials that demonstrated improvement in patients with both optic nerve and postchiasmal lesions after training with their computerized system.

hemisphere and recruitment of likely extrastriate (V3a, hMT+) areas on the damaged left side. (*Reprinted from* Das A, Huxlin KR. New approaches to visual rehabilitation for cortical blindness: outcomes and putative mechanisms. Neuroscientist 2010;16:374–87; with permission.)

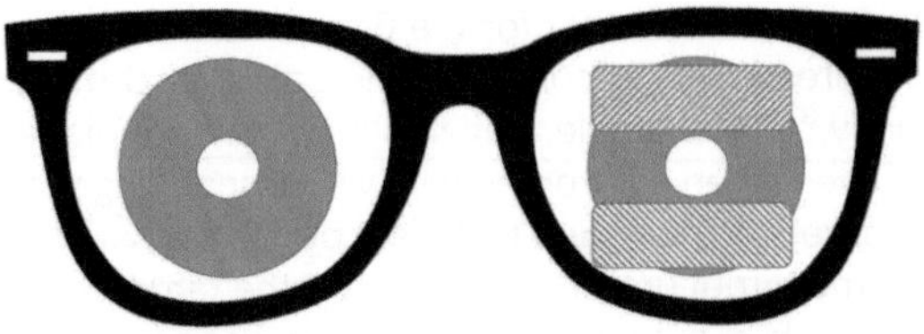

Fig. 4. Obliquely oriented high-power Fresnel prism to expand the visual field. The placement of prism over the left spectacle lens, as in this example, would be done to increase awareness of the left hemifield in a patient with a left homonymous hemianopia. The commercially available prisms (Chadwick Optical, Souderton, PA) are typically 57 prism diopters and expand the field by about 30°.

The original NovaVision training protocol[9] required patients to train for 1 hour daily (2 30 minute sessions), 6 times a week, for 6 months. Each patient's scotoma was mapped during an initial diagnostic evaluation, and the software determined areas for potential improvement. In subsequent therapeutic sessions, patients sat in a dark room, positioned at a set distance from a computer screen. They were asked to fixate continuously on a central target, after which hundreds of suprathreshold stimuli were presented in succession at the transition zone between the intact visual field and the scotoma. The patients pressed a key every time they detected a stimulus. The system monitored fixation by requiring patients to respond within 500 ms to color changes in the central target.

Patients who participated in the initial studies had damage to either the optic nerve or the primary visual cortex, and, importantly, the patient's injury occurred more than 12 months before the study to minimize the potential confounding effect of spontaneous recovery. Baseline visual field assessment and outcome measures were done using a campimetric system termed high-resolution perimetry (HRP), with secondary outcome measures done using Tübingen automated perimetry (TAP). (These and other perimetry methods are discussed in more detail elsewhere in this article). The authors reported statistically significant improvement in stimulus detection in the hemianopic field, and a shift in the transition zone of 5 to 6° among VRT-trained patients. This transition zone shift represents an enlargement of the visual field and a decrease in the size of the scotoma as determined by HRP. When examined by TAP, subjects with optic nerve lesions (but not visual cortex lesions) showed a reduction in the size of their scotoma; the border shift in cortical lesions was 0.43°, and in optic nerve lesions 2.1° as compared with the 4.9 and 5.8° seen with HRP. Finally, questionnaires revealed subjective improvement in 72.2% of patients trained with VRT, as compared with 16.6% of controls[9] (**Fig. 5**).

Although enticing because of the potential clinical benefit and apparent plasticity of the visual system, VRT was controversial from the outset owing to concerns regarding the validity of the studies purporting its value. Specifically, critics suggested that eye movements during training and subsequent campimetric testing were not recorded or well controlled for. It was postulated that patients developed strategies while using NovaVision similar to those acquired naturally after homonymous visual loss, as described.[27] Editorials such as those by Horton[34] claimed that Sabel and his group did not report fixation losses, false positives, and false negatives, and that their use of blind spot monitoring was inadequate to detect small saccades.

The assessment of any potential visual restoration technique ultimately must rely on a reproducible and appropriate perimetric method. Standard automated perimetry tests points that are separated by 6° (when the central 24°–30° is being evaluated) and

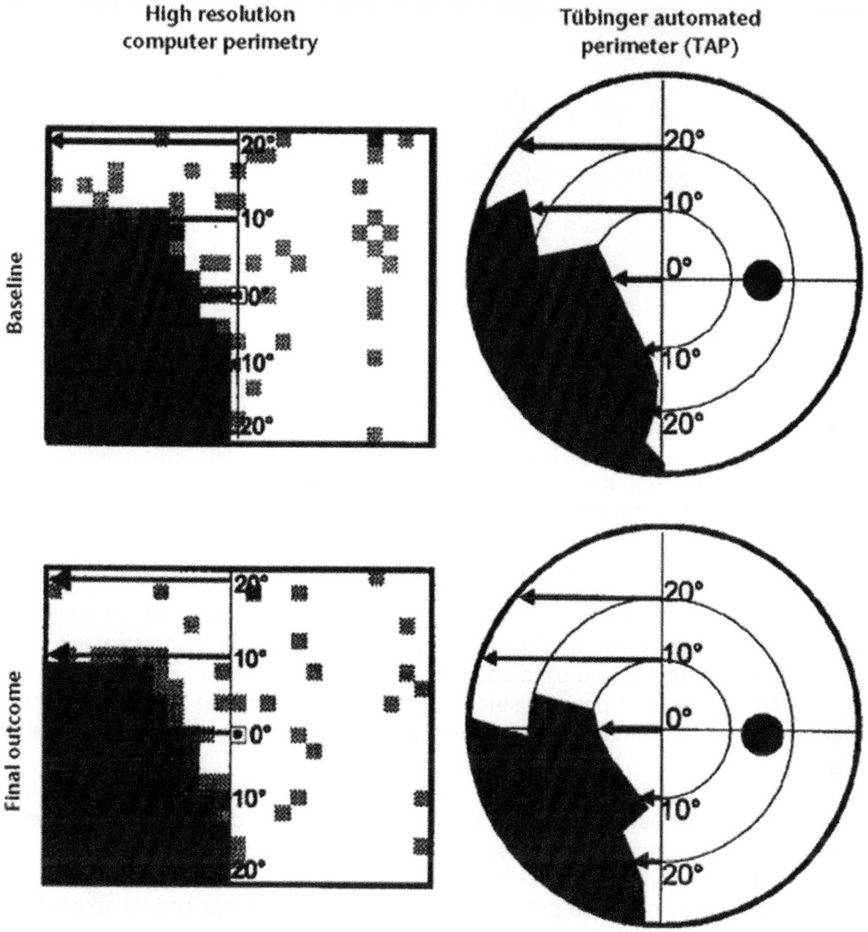

Fig. 5. Visual field expansion with vision restoration therapy, demonstrated with both high-resolution perimetry and Tübingen automated perimetry. (*Reprinted from* Kasten E, Wüst S, Behrens-Baumann W, et al. Computer-based training for the treatment of partial blindness. Nat Med 1998;4:1083–7; with permission.)

does not detect more subtle changes. The test relies on blind spot monitoring to control for fixation losses, which in a typical patient result from loss of concentration and will be evidenced as a large saccade or drift away from the intended target. HRP, a system developed by Sabel's group, creates a map of the visual field and scotoma using 3 to 5 stimuli of 150 ms in duration in a 25- by 20-point grid, which spans the central 42° of the visual field on the horizontal axis and 32° on the vertical axis.[9] Patients fixate on a central star, and press a key when they see a stimulus (within 750 ms). As described, fixation is not recorded, but is determined by random changes in the color of the central fixation star, for which the patients have to press a key within 500 ms. The HRP system then creates a grayscale map of the intact visual field (white), the scotoma (black), and the transition zone (gray) based on the percentage of correct responses (**Fig. 6**).

TAP is a more conventional method of threshold perimetry, akin to the standard perimetry systems in widespread clinical use. Fixation in TAP is maintained by

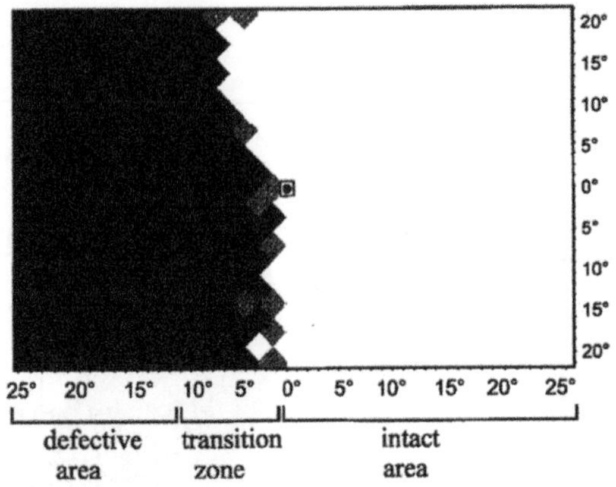

Fig. 6. Damaged visual field (*black*), intact visual field (*white*), and transition zone (*gray*) in which visual restoration therapy is directed in an attempt to stimulate anticipated residual function. (*Reprinted from* Kasten E, Wüst S, Behrens-Baumann W, et al. Computer-based training for the treatment of partial blindness. Nat Med 1998;4:1083–7; with permission.)

presenting a stimulus in the center of the fixation square at random intervals, and the percentage of correct hits in the fixation square is recorded. This method stands in contrast with the blind spot stimulation used by commercial instruments to monitor fixation, in which response to a blind spot stimulus is recorded as a fixation loss. In the original VRT studies, 191 points distributed up to 30° eccentric to fixation were evaluated with threshold stimulation.[35] Of note, HRP evaluates 500 points within the same area.

Scanning laser ophthalmoscope (SLO) perimetry is another visual field assessment (not used in the original VRT studies). In this system, gaze is directed into a red rectangle with a small central fixation cross. Three black dots of varying configuration and interdot distance are presented on a bright background in various retinal locations for a short time (ie, 120 ms). The patient then describes the number and location of the dots. SLO is different from TAP and HRP in that the retina is visualized in real time during the testing, so if the patient's fixation is interrupted by a saccade, the examiner can discard the result and repeat the same stimulus once fixation is maintained.[36]

As mentioned, Horton's criticism of the original VRT data in part focused on HRP's inadequate control for quick saccades into the blind hemifield. Specifically, Horton stated that:

> *Patients with homonymous field defects compensate by making frequent saccades toward their scotoma in an effort to maintain surveillance of blind regions in their visual fields. It is notoriously difficult to control fixation in such subjects. During visual restoration therapy, fixation is monitored by randomly changing the color of a 0.75° fixation light from bright green to yellow, whereupon the subject is required to respond within 500 ms by pressing a button. The problem with this technique is that the color transition is so easy to detect that it does not require foveal vision. Patients soon learn that they can sneak 5° saccades into their blind hemifield, and still detect a change in the color of the fixation monitoring light. Hence, the mean 5° improvement in the visual field.*[34]

In other words, patients may be trained inadvertently to quickly scan parts of their blind hemifield and still be able to detect a color change of the fixation marker, which would make them seem to have field enlargement when assessed by HRP. A potentially serious flaw in the original VRT studies, namely the use of the same system for training and outcome assessment, may have led to the mischaracterization of these scanning saccades as true visual field expansion and improvement.

To address these concerns, Reinhard and colleagues[36] evaluated 17 patients with homonymous field defects resulting from postchiasmal injury at least 1 year after their injury using SLO perimetry after the standard 6-month protocol described in the initial VRT studies. This study showed drastically different results from the original HRP-evaluated cohort: only 1 patient showed minimal improvement of their visual field by slightly more than 1°, and only in 1 eye. Furthermore, Schreiber and colleagues[35] reported TAP data from 16 of the same 17 patients and concluded that only 2 patients demonstrated greater than 2° of visual field enlargement, and in both patients this change was monocular, making central plasticity an unlikely explanation for such improvement. An editorial back-and-forth was initiated by Horton's initial commentary, and is instructive in demonstrating the extent of the controversy.

- Sabel and colleagues[37] responded that:
  - HRP and TAP data obtained concurrently with the negative SLO study, respectively, showed:
    - Positive changes in the scotoma border,[35] and
    - An average field enlargement of 1.73°, with an improved percentage of detected stimuli.[38]
  - Conflicting data can be explained in several ways:
    - HRP is superior to TAP and SLO because of relative ease of use of HRP;
    - TAP data should be reported as number of misses instead of number of hits, and that VRT causes a decrease in the number of misses on average[38];
    - SLO misinterprets border zone to be scotoma, unlike HRP, implying that HRP is more sensitive in detecting improvements after training; or
    - Eye movements are unlikely to have contributed to the positive HRP data given that patients showed excellent fixation using the other perimetry methods, even after VRT.
- In response, Horton[39] contended that:
  - Blind spot position is an imperfect method for detecting small breaks in fixation, and that it cannot be used at all in patients with temporal hemianopia and
  - SLO is in fact more sensitive than HRP because it characterizes relative defects as normal.
- Sabel[40] rejoined that:
  - Fixation losses do not explain the positive HRP data, as verified by a subsequently published study using visual tracking technology to ensure that saccadic eye movements were not changed after training,[41]
  - The differences in the HRP and SLO data is owing to the greater task difficulty of SLO, and
  - SLO is in fact less sensitive that HRP because it characterizes relative defects as blind.

More recently, larger clinical trials to assess VRT have been undertaken. A trial by Mueller and colleagues[42] evaluated 302 patients with a similar protocol to the original VRT studies, and performed both pretraining and posttraining perimetry using HRP. A subset of these patients (n = 69) were also tested with standard perimetry and subjective questionnaires, and a smaller subset had eye movements tracked with an infrared eye-tracking system (n = 20). In this study, the primary outcome was the percentage of "hits," or correct response to the suprathreshold stimuli delivered by HRP. The study found that after training, the number of hits increased by an average of 9.7

($P < .001$), and the majority of these were owing to detection of stimuli in the defective part of the visual field. The average shift in the visual border was found to be 4.9° in these patients, consistent with the initial VRT trial. In those patients also tested with conventional perimetry, the number of false hits decreased, and the results were significantly correlated ($P < .001$). Interestingly, the paper also showed that the only factor influencing outcome was the size of the residual vision. Patients with greater areas of residual vision also showed greater improvement in their visual fields, leading the authors to speculate that these patients had more neurons in those residual areas that had the potential to be activated by VRT. This study, however, was not placebo controlled, unlike the original VRT studies. Furthermore, data on the subset of patients evaluated with SLO perimetry was not presented. An additional confounding factor was introduced by the inclusion of patients with prechiasmatic disorders, in whom cortical plasticity would not be a plausible mechanism for recovery.

In contrast, more recent evidence suggests that VRT can be effective when patients with prechiasmatic disorders are evaluated. Building on the results as presented, Sabel and Gudlin[43] published a prospective, double-blind RCT assessing the effects of VRT in patients with visual field deficits owing to glaucoma, showing improvements in these patients as well. In this study, 30 patients with glaucoma underwent VRT for 3 months. The primary outcome measure was detection accuracy by HRP, and eye tracking technology was used to control for breaks in fixation. The study showed a significant increase in the HRP detection rate in the VRT group as compared with controls ($P < .007$), although improvement was greatly variable among the patients. About one-third of patients showed no improvement, one-third showed moderate improvement, and one-third achieved substantial improvement. Interestingly, detection accuracy was not improved significantly when measured by standard perimetry (although the trend was toward improvement). In contrast with Mueller's data,[42] accuracy was not significantly greater in patients with larger areas of residual vision. Finally, patients did not show a difference in mean gaze position and position variability after training as compared with baseline, indicating that there was no change in fixation quality to explain the improvements seen.

Although the focus of this review is the data and controversy regarding VRT, it is important to note that a myriad of other attempts at visual field restoration have been undertaken. For example, 1 small study evaluated 2 patients trained with a flickering letter identification task and showed that, after intensive training, flicker sensitivity and letter recognition in the trained areas improved significantly.[17] This indicates the possibility of training-responsive improvements in previously hemianopic regions of the visual field, although without enlargements in the visual field size by perimetric measures. Other studies have compared similar training with explorative saccade training and found the latter to be superior.[44] Yet another small study used intensive training in direction discrimination in patients with V1 damage, showing improved ability to discriminate motion, as well as improved contrast sensitivity and extraction of motion signal from noise.[18] In addition, other data indicate that combined methods of training, for example, transcranial direct current stimulation in combination with VRT, may be more effective than 1 method alone.[45,46]

SUMMARY

VRT remains a controversial yet intriguing subject, both because there are clear published data regarding its benefit in visual field improvement and because of the remaining nagging questions as to the validity of that data and the clinical benefit of such training, especially in the face of the cost and time involved in such training. This is especially true because there are consistent animal data demonstrating improvement after training of the visual system, and there are a myriad of proposed mechanisms that could underlie visual field improvements. In addition, because of the well-demonstrated phenomenon of spontaneous improvement after visual field damage in the initial weeks to months after injury, studies have recruited patients remote from their time of injury to avoid confounding of their data. What this means, however, is that there is no information at all regarding whether early intervention may be of benefit, as has clearly been shown in rehabilitation after damage in other parts of the central nervous system. In addition, studies seem to indicate that improvement after training is specific to the type of training performed (ie, motion discrimination training results in improvements in that and closely related tasks only), and there is question as to whether such improvements truly translate to clinically significant improvement for patients.[13,46] Again, this is a critical consideration given that these interventions may be quite expensive, making it even more vital to ensure that the results obtained are both valid and clinically significant.

In sum, there are theoretic underpinnings, animal data, and human experience to suggest that there is a large amount of potential for plasticity in the visual system, despite the gestalt to the contrary. Moreover, this plasticity seems to be highly dependent on the extent and location of damage, as well as on the training mechanism used to exploit it and the perimetric methods used to assess it. Although multiple studies have showed statistically significant effects after various training protocols, controversy remains as to their validity and applicability in clinical practice. Neither VRT nor other researched methods of visual system training have led to standardized approaches to visual rehabilitation in patients with visual field defects, indicating that larger and more targeted studies are still needed to determine the best approach to the patient with a new visual field defect in clinical practice.

REFERENCES

1. Han L, Law-Gibson D, Reding M. Key neurological impairments influence function-related group outcomes after stroke. Stroke 2002;33:1920–4.
2. Patel AT, Duncan PW, Lai SM, et al. The relation between impairments and functional outcomes poststroke. Arch Phys Med Rehabil 2000;81:1357–63.
3. Pambakian A, Currie J, Kennard C. Rehabilitation strategies for patients with homonymous visual field defects. J Neuroophthalmol 2005;25:136–42.
4. Pambakian AL, Kennard C. Can visual function be restored in patients with homonymous hemianopia? Br J Ophthalmol 1997;81:324–8.
5. Huxlin KR, Williams JM, Price T. A neurochemical signature of visual recovery after extrastriate cortical damage in the adult cat. J Comp Neurol 2008;508:45–61.
6. Huxlin KR, Pasternak T. Training-induced recovery of visual motion perception after extrastriate cortical damage in the adult cat. Cereb Cortex 2004;14:81–90.
7. Dilks DD, Serences JT, Rosenau BJ, et al. Human adult cortical reorganization and consequent visual distortion. J Neurosci 2007;27:9585–94.
8. Huxlin KR. Perceptual plasticity in damaged adult visual systems. Vision Res 2008;48:2154–66.
9. Kasten E, Wüst S, Behrens-Baumann W, et al. Computer-based training for the treatment of partial blindness. Nat Med 1998;4:1083–7.
10. Strand T, Asplund K, Eriksson S, et al. Stroke unit care–who benefits? Comparisons with general medical care in relation to prognostic indicators on admission. Stroke 1986;17:377–81.
11. Minematsu K. Acute ischemic stroke. Rinsho Shinkeigaku 2003;43:796–8 [in Japanese].

12. Turner-Stokes L, Pick A, Nair A, et al. Multi-disciplinary rehabilitation for acquired brain injury in adults of working age. Cochrane Database Syst Rev 2015;12: CD004170.
13. Das A, Huxlin KR. New approaches to visual rehabilitation for cortical blindness: outcomes and putative mechanisms. Neuroscientist 2010;16:374–87.
14. Goodwin D. Homonymous hemianopia: challenges and solutions. Clin Ophthalmol 2014;8:1919–27.
15. Zhang X, Kedar S, Lynn MJ, et al. Homonymous hemianopias: clinical-anatomic correlations in 904 cases. Neurology 2006;66:906–10.
16. Zhang X, Kedar S, Lynn MJ, et al. Natural history of homonymous hemianopia. Neurology 2006;66:901–5.
17. Raninen A, Vanni S, Hyvärinen L, et al. Temporal sensitivity in a hemianopic visual field can be improved by long-term training using flicker stimulation. J Neurol Neurosurg Psychiatr 2007;78:66–73.
18. Huxlin KR, Martin T, Kelly K, et al. Perceptual relearning of complex visual motion after V1 damage in humans. J Neurosci 2009;29:3981–91.
19. Cowey A, Weiskrantz L. A perimetric study of visual field defects in monkeys. Q J Exp Psychol 1963;15:91–115.
20. Mohler CW, Wurtz RH. Role of striate cortex and superior colliculus in visual guidance of saccadic eye movements in monkeys. J Neurophysiol 1977;40:74–94.
21. Schiller PH. The effects of V4 and middle temporal (MT) area lesions on visual performance in the rhesus monkey. Vis Neurosci 1993;10:717–46.
22. Merigan WH, Pham HA. V4 lesions in macaques affect both single- and multiple-viewpoint shape discriminations. Vis Neurosci 1998;15:359–67.
23. Poppelreuter W. Die psychischen Schädingungen durch Kopfschuss im Kriege 1914/16: mit besonderer Berücksichtigung der pathopsychologischen, pädagogischen, gewerblichen und sozialen Beziehungen. Band I: Die Störungen der niederen un höheren Sehleistungen durch Verletzungen des Okzipitalhirns. Leipzig (Germany): L. Voss; 1917.
24. Luria AR. Restoration of function after brain injury. Oxford: Macmillan; 1963.
25. Zihl J, Cramon von D. Visual field recovery from scotoma in patients with postgeniculate damage. A review of 55 cases. Brain 1985;108(Pt 2):335–65.
26. Bach-y-Rita P. Controlling variables eliminates hemianopsia rehabilitation results. Behav Brain Sci 1983;6:448.
27. Pelak VS, Dubin M, Whitney E. Homonymous hemianopia: a critical analysis of optical devices, compensatory training, and novavision. Curr Treat Options Neurol 2007;9:41–7.
28. Zihl J. Recovery of visual functions in patients with cerebral blindness. Effect of specific practice with saccadic localization. Exp Brain Res 1981;44:159–69.
29. Kerkhoff G. Neurovisual rehabilitation: recent developments and future directions. J Neurol Neurosurg Psychiatr 2000;68:691–706.
30. Rossi PW, Kheyfets S, Reding MJ. Fresnel prisms improve visual perception in stroke patients with homonymous hemianopia or unilateral visual neglect. Neurology 1990;40:1597–9.
31. Peli E. Field expansion for homonymous hemianopia by optically induced peripheral exotropia. Optom Vis Sci 2000;77:453–64.
32. Cowey A. Perimetric study of field defects in monkeys after cortical and retinal ablations. Q J Exp Psychol 1967;19:232–45.
33. Zihl J. Zur Behandlung von Patienten mit homonymen Gesichtsfeldstörungen. Z Neuropsychol 1990;2:95–101.

34. Horton JC. Disappointing results from nova vision's visual restoration therapy. Br J Ophthalmol 2005;89:1–2.
35. Schreiber A, Vonthein R, Reinhard J, et al. Effect of visual restitution training on absolute homonymous scotomas. Neurology 2006;67:143–5.
36. Reinhard J, Schreiber A, Schiefer U, et al. Does visual restitution training change absolute homonymous visual field defects? A fundus controlled study. Br J Ophthalmol 2005;89:30–5.
37. Sabel BA, Kenkel S, Kasten E. Vision restoration therapy. Br J Ophthalmol 2005; 89:522–4.
38. Sabel BA, Kenkel S, Kasten E. Vision restoration therapy (VRT) efficacy as assessed by comparative perimetric analysis and subjective questionnaires. Restor Neurol Neurosci 2004;22:399–420.
39. Horton JC. Vision restoration therapy: confounded by eye movements. Br J Ophthalmol 2005;89:792–4.
40. Sabel BA. Vision restoration therapy and raising red flags too early. Br J Ophthalmol 2006;90:659–60.
41. Kasten E, Bunzenthal U, Sabel BA. Visual field recovery after vision restoration therapy (VRT) is independent of eye movements: an eye tracker study. Behav Brain Res 2006;175:18–26.
42. Mueller I, Mast H, Sabel BA. Recovery of visual field defects: a large clinical observational study using vision restoration therapy. Restor Neurol Neurosci 2007;25:563–72.
43. Sabel BA, Gudlin J. Vision restoration training for glaucoma: a randomized clinical trial. JAMA Ophthalmol 2014;132:381–9.
44. Roth T, Sokolov AN, Messias A, et al. Comparing explorative saccade and flicker training in hemianopia: a randomized controlled study. Neurology 2009;72: 324–31.
45. Plow EB, Obretenova SN, Halko MA, et al. Combining visual rehabilitative training and noninvasive brain stimulation to enhance visual function in patients with hemianopia: a comparative case study. PM R 2011;3:825–35.
46. Miller NR, Subramanian PS. Should visual restoration therapy be used in patients with visual field loss? J Neuroophthalmol 2015;35(3):319–22.

Update on Idiopathic Intracranial Hypertension

Michael Wall, MD

KEYWORDS

- Idiopathic intracranial hypertension • Pseudotumor cerebri • Acetazolamide
- Optical coherence tomography

KEY POINTS

- Acetazolamide when used in patients with idiopathic intracranial hypertension (IIH) with mild visual loss produces a modest improvement in perimetric mean deviation on visual field testing over 6 months. The improvement is much greater in patients with moderate-to high-grade papilledema.
- Acetazolamide has its greatest effect on visual field function and papilledema in the first month of escalating dosage.
- In the IIH treatment trial, treatment failure was much less common in the acetazolamide-plus-diet group compared with the placebo-plus-diet group, and risk factors for treatment failure were presence of high-grade papilledema and lower visual acuity measures at baseline.
- Positive acetazolamide-related effects on quality of life seemed to be primarily mediated by improvements in visual field, neck pain, pulsatile tinnitus, and dizziness/vertigo that outweighed the side effects of acetazolamide.
- High cerebrospinal fluid pressure decreases the size of the entire dural sinus tree and also results in increasing size of skull foramen, canals, and ostia.

Idiopathic intracranial hypertension (IIH) is a disorder of overweight women in the childbearing age characterized by increased intracranial pressure with its associated signs and symptoms in alert and oriented patients. Neuroimaging and cerebrospinal fluid (CSF) analysis is normal except for increased intracranial pressure and its associated symptoms and signs. Also, no secondary cause of intracranial hypertension is apparent. This set of criteria comprises the modified Dandy criteria (**Box 1**). In the last 3 years, there has been an explosion of publications on IIH, with a PubMed search revealing more than 500 articles. In this review, the authors discuss the most important of these articles, especially those generated from the Idiopathic Intracranial Hypertension Treatment Trial (IIHT).

Before 3 years ago, a Cochrane review concluded: "*There is insufficient information to generate an evidence-based management strategy for idiopathic intracranial*

Disclosure statement: No relevant disclosures.
University of Iowa College of Medicine, Veterans Administration Hospital, Iowa City, IA 52242, USA
E-mail address: michael-wall@uiowa.edu

Neurol Clin 35 (2017) 45–57
http://dx.doi.org/10.1016/j.ncl.2016.08.004 neurologic.theclinics.com

Box 1
The modified Dandy criteria for idiopathic intracranial hypertension used in the Idiopathic Intracranial Hypertension Treatment Trial

1. Signs and symptoms of increased intracranial pressure
2. Absence of localizing findings on neurologic examination
3. Absence of deformity, displacement, or obstruction of the ventricular system and otherwise normal neurodiagnostic studies, except for evidence of increased CSF pressure (>200 mm water) (Abnormal neuroimaging except for empty sella turcica, optic nerve sheath with filled-out CSF spaces, and smooth-walled non–flow-related venous sinus stenosis 106 should lead to another diagnosis.)
4. Awake and alert
5. No other cause of increased intracranial pressure present

hypertension. There is inadequate information regarding which treatments are truly beneficial and which are potentially harmful. Properly designed and executed trials are needed."[1] In April 2014, the IIHTT results were published in the *Journal of the American Medical Association*.[2] This trial gave us the first evidenced-based approach relating to a protocol that significantly improved visual function in IIH.

THE IDIOPATHIC INTRACRANIAL HYPERTENSION TREATMENT TRIAL

In 1897, Quincke reported the first cases of IIH shortly after he introduced the lumbar puncture into medicine. It was named *pseudotumor cerebri* in 1904 but was not well delineated clinically until the 1940s when cerebral angiography was added to pneumoencephalography to identify cases of cerebral mass lesions. Foley coined the term *benign intracranial hypertension* in 1955; but reports from the 1980s demonstrated a high incidence of visual loss,[3,4] and the term *benign* is no longer appropriate.

Lubow and Kuhr[5] reported a series of patients with IIH, many of whom were treated successfully with acetazolamide and weight reduction.[6] The latter, another mainstay of medical therapy, was further shown to be a viable treatment by others. Gücer and Viernstein[7] used intracranial pressure monitoring and showed gradual CSF pressure reduction in patients receiving acetazolamide once they reached a dosage of 3 to 4 g/d. These uncontrolled studies were the basis for using acetazolamide in the maximally tolerated dosage to treat IIH.

The IIHTT is a multicenter, double-blind, randomized placebo-controlled study of acetazolamide in subjects with IIH with mild visual loss.[2,8] The trial structure and flow is found in **Fig. 1**. All subjects received a lifestyle modification program that included weight reduction with a low-sodium diet. The purpose of the trial was to determine the effect of acetazolamide in reducing or reversing visual loss after 6 months of treatment.

Subjects needed to meet the modified Dandy criteria for IIH and be aged 18 to 60 years. They needed to have reproducible mild visual loss (−2 to −7 dB perimetric mean deviation [PMD]). Participants needed to have bilateral papilledema, have an elevated CSF opening pressure, be untreated with regard to IIH, and have no secondary cause of increased intracranial pressure present.

Subjects were randomly assigned to receive a supervised lifestyle modification program that included a low-sodium weight-reduction diet either with acetazolamide or with matching placebo. The initial dosage of the study drug was 4 tablets daily in 2 divided doses, followed by dosage increases of 1 tablet every week up to a maximum

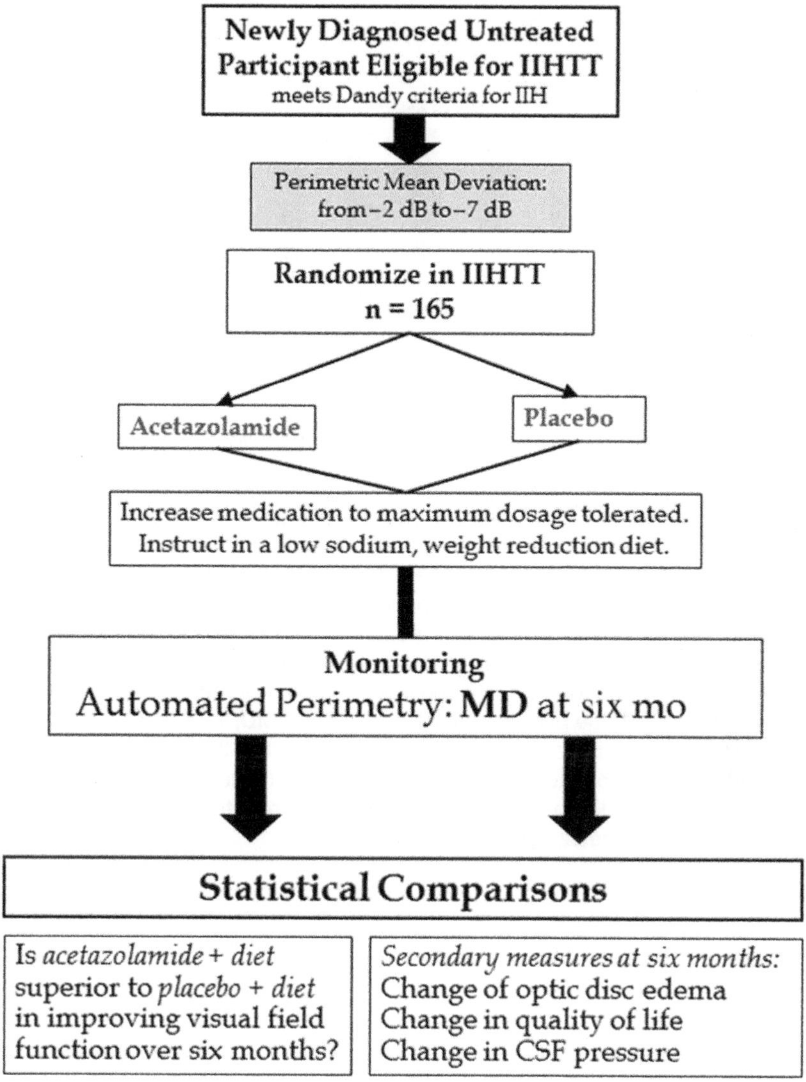

Fig. 1. Clinical trial structure for the IIHTT. MD, mean deviation.

dosage of 4 g/d for participants receiving acetazolamide. The dosage escalation was stopped if the participant's papilledema grade became less than 1 in both eyes and the PMD improved to −1 dB or better in each eye, unless the presence of other symptoms, such as headache or pulse synchronous tinnitus, suggested that the dosage escalation continue.

In the IIHTT, 161 women and 4 men were enrolled with an average age of 29.0 years (range 18–52 years). **Fig. 2** shows the frequency of symptoms at baseline. The baseline characteristics were comparable in the two treatment groups; additional baseline information is published elsewhere.[9] There were 7 participants whose vision worsened to meet the end point of treatment failure in the trial, with 6 treatment failures in the placebo group and 1 in the acetazolamide group (P = .06).[2,10] Patients with IIH with

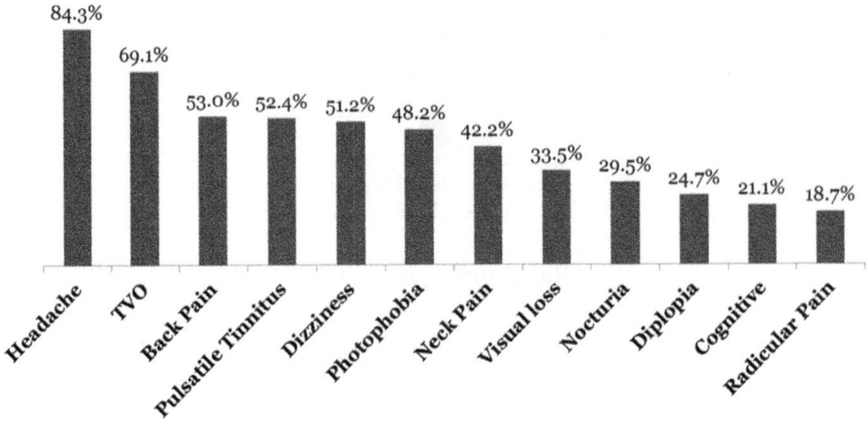

Fig. 2. Frequency of symptoms at study entry. TVO, transient visual obscurations.

high-grade papilledema, daily transient visual obscurations, and decreased visual acuity at baseline were more likely to experience treatment failure. Patients with this profile should be treated more aggressively.[10]

Both treatment groups experienced improvement in PMD over time in the study eye (**Fig. 3**), with the mean improvement in the acetazolamide group being significantly larger than that in the placebo group at month 6 ($P = .05$).[2] Most of the improvement related to acetazolamide took place in the first month of the intervention. Interestingly, the treatment effect on the primary outcome variable, PMD, was substantially greater (2.27 dB) in those with a baseline papilledema grade of 3 to 5 than in those with a baseline papilledema grade of 1 to 2 (−0.67 dB).[2] Therefore, those with moderate- to high-grade papilledema are the patients who benefit most from treatment with maximally tolerated dosages of acetazolamide.

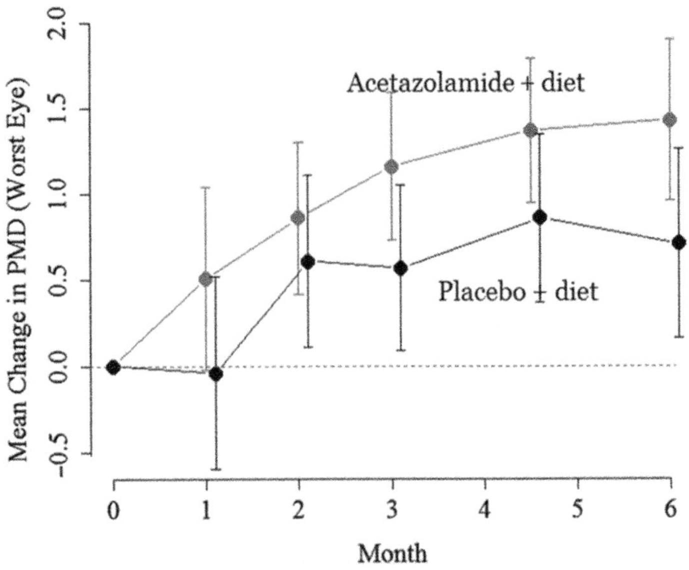

Fig. 3. Perimetric mean deviation change over 6 months in the IIHTT.

Visual acuity was mildly decreased at baseline (**Fig. 4**). This finding is especially notable when one factors in that visual acuity should be at least 20/15 in this age group. With treatment, acuity improved modestly; but the change was not statistically significant at 6 months. Perimetry is a much better measure to use to follow patients with IIH than visual acuity.

The visual field defects found at baseline were typical for IIH.[11] The prototype defect was an enlarged blind spot coupled with an inferior nasal nerve fiber bundle defect (**Fig. 5**). However, there was usually mild loss across the visual field; although in the more central portions of the visual field, the loss did not reach the 95th percentile cut-off for abnormality.

There was significant improvement in the Frisén papilledema grade associated with acetazolamide treatment in the study eye and in the fellow eye (**Fig. 6**). As with mean deviation, most of the benefit from acetazolamide was in the first month.

Acetazolamide-treated participants also experienced significant improvement in quality-of-life measures, including the Visual Functioning Questionnaire-25 total score and its 10-item neuro-ophthalmic supplement as well as the 36-Item Short Form Physical Component Summary and Mental Component Summary scores. Positive acetazolamide-related effects on quality of life seemed to be primarily mediated by improvements in visual field, neck pain, pulsatile tinnitus, and dizziness/vertigo that outweighed the side effects of acetazolamide. No significant acetazolamide treatment effects were noted with respect to headache disability (Headache Impact Test-6 total score) as both treatment groups had improved HIT scores. This finding may be due to subjects having concomitant analgesic rebound headaches, and both groups received additional headache medications (usually naproxen sodium or low-dosage amitriptyline).

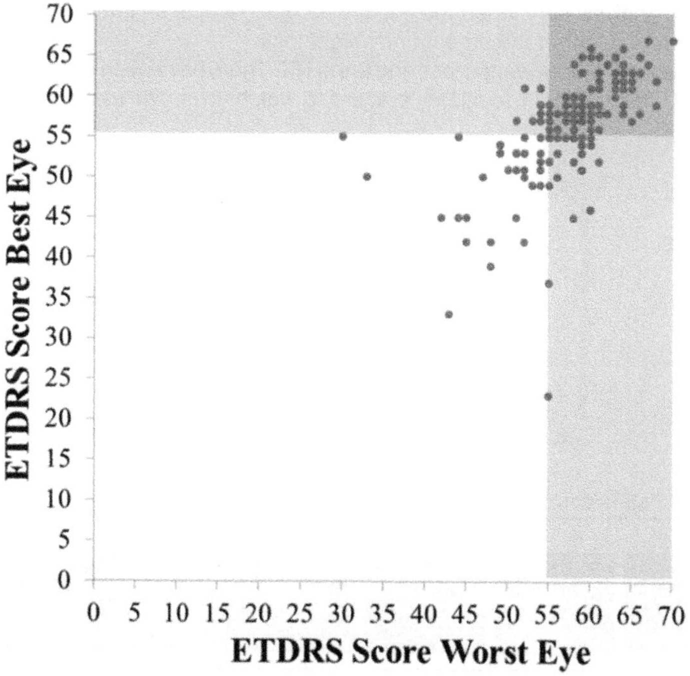

Fig. 4. ETDRS score of worst eye plotted against best eye. Shaded areas indicate vision of 20/20 or better.

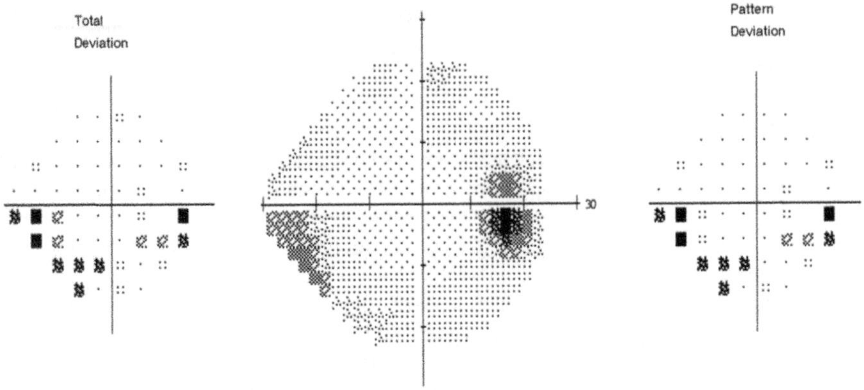

Fig. 5. The prototype visual field defect in patients with IIH with mild loss: the inferior nasal arcuate defect. Not the arcuate pattern of the abnormal test locations flagged on the Total Deviation plot.

With regard to CSF pressure, the decrease in CSF pressure in the acetazolamide group was −112.3 mm H_2O and was −52.4 mm H_2O in the placebo group giving a treatment effect of −59.9 H_2O ($P = .002$; **Fig. 7**).

Clinical improvement in IIH has been reported to be associated with about 6% weight loss.[12] Participants on acetazolamide lost more weight over 6 months (mean −7.50 kg, from 107.72 kg to 100.22 kg) than those on placebo (mean −3.45 kg, from 107.72 kg to 104.27 kg) (treatment effect −4.05, $P<.001$). Acetazolamide also led to reductions in waist circumference and systolic and diastolic blood pressure.[2] A mediation analysis concluded the effect of acetazolamide on improved visual function was *independent* of the amount of weight loss.

Misconceptions about weight loss and the IIHTT: There have been some misconceptions about what the IIHTT found with regard to weight loss. *The trial did not compare*

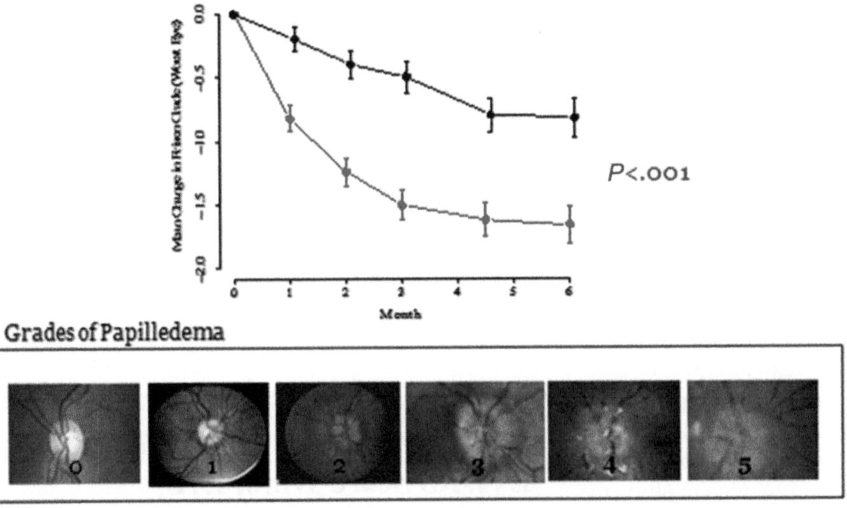

Fig. 6. Change in papilledema grade in the eye with the worst initial mean deviation over 6 months.

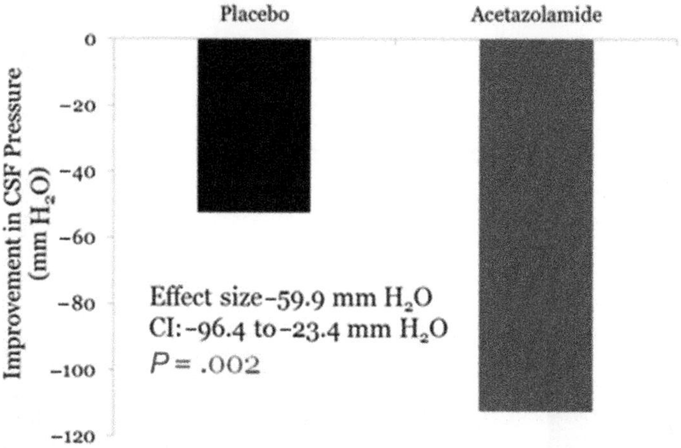

Fig. 7. Reduction in CSF pressure over 6 months in the placebo and acetazolamide groups in the IIHTT. CI, confidence interval.

acetazolamide with weight loss. It compared acetazolamide with placebo in the setting where all were receiving a weight loss intervention. The IIHTT cannot estimate an effect of weight loss, as the authors did not design their study to determine the effect of weight loss. The authors did *not* find that both acetazolamide and weight loss improved visual field function; acetazolamide improved visual field function in a setting of weight reduction. Weight loss might have improved vision as well, but the authors cannot determine this without studying people who did not have a weight loss intervention.

The authors also did not show what percent weight loss is required to have resolution of IIH. They do not know if these people would have had resolution even without a weight loss intervention because they did not have this control group. Also, the authors do not know if acetazolamide would work the same way if given in a setting without a concurrent weight loss intervention.

In the trial, 48 eyes from 35 subjects met the visual field criteria for possible treatment failure. Seven subjects were found to have treatment failure. On retest, these other subjects had their PMD return to acceptable limits. Four of the variable performance subjects had large changes on retest and were reviewed by the adjudication committee and determined to be "performance failures" (temporary substantial worsening of PMD).[13]

Adverse events that occurred in greater than 5% of study participants did not cause permanent morbidity, including 9 serious adverse events.[14] Although paresthesia, dysgeusia, vomiting, diarrhea, nausea, and fatigue were higher in the acetazolamide group than in the placebo group, quality-of-life measures were superior in the acetazolamide group. A mild decrease in mean potassium level was also seen with acetazolamide, but this did not require potassium supplementation in any participants. No significant changes in sodium levels or in liver function tests were apparent with acetazolamide except for the case noted earlier.

Average compliance (as measured by counts of dispensed and returned pills) was 89% in the acetazolamide group and 93% in the placebo group. The mean (standard deviation) dose of study medication that participants were taking at the conclusion of their participation was 2.5 g (1.5 g) in the acetazolamide group and 3.5 g (1.1 g) in the placebo group (**Fig. 8**).

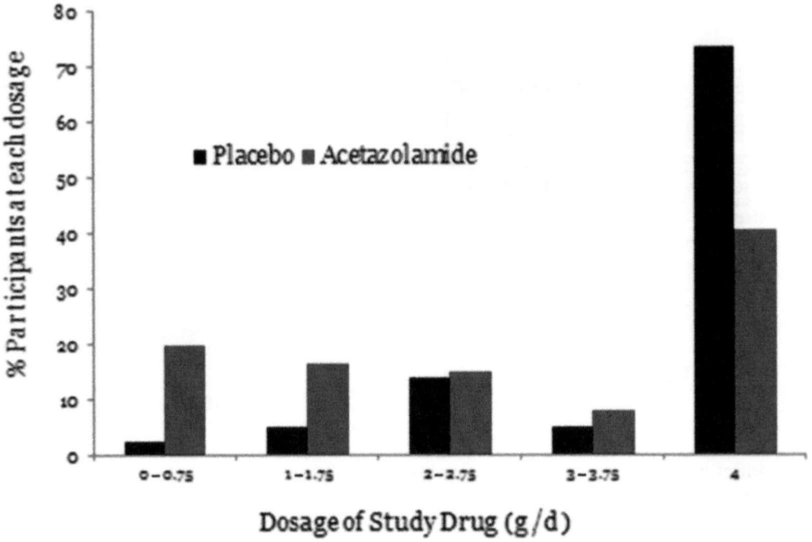

Fig. 8. Final dosage reached for placebo and acetazolamide subjects in the IIHTT.

A limitation of the study is the 19% withdrawal rate, although the frequency of and reasons for withdrawal were similar in the two treatment groups. This rate may be due, in part, to the intensity of the visit schedule. More subjects on acetazolamide than on placebo discontinued treatment, most of whom completed follow-up, which may have attenuated the estimated treatment effect.

The results of the IIHTT, a multicenter, randomized, double-masked, placebo-controlled study of acetazolamide in subjects with mild visual loss, demonstrate improvements in visual field function, papilledema grade, and quality-of-life measures (**Box 2**). The authors recommend using the maximally tolerated dosage, up to 4 g daily, of acetazolamide with a low-sodium, weight-reduction diet in patients with IIH with mild visual loss.

What Have We Learned from the Idiopathic Intracranial Hypertension Treatment Trial?

- Acetazolamide, when used in subjects with IIH with mild visual loss, produces a modest improvement in PMD over 6 months. The improvement is much greater in subjects with moderate- to high-grade papilledema.
- Acetazolamide has its greatest effect on visual field function and papilledema in the first month of escalating dosage.

Box 2
The Idiopathic Intracranial Hypertension Treatment Trial showed statistically significant effects of acetazolamide to

- Improve visual field function
- Decrease papilledema grade
- Improve quality-of-life measures
- Decrease CSF pressure

- Acetazolamide-plus-diet subjects lost twice as much weight as placebo-plus-diet subjects, but the acetazolamide effect on PMD was independent of the weight loss.
- Treatment failure was much less common in the acetazolamide-plus-diet group compared with the placebo-plus-diet group, and risk factors for treatment failure were presence of high-grade papilledema and lower ETDRS (Early Treatment Diabetic Retinopathy Study) visual acuity measures at baseline.
- Many IIHTT subjects tolerated maximal dosages of acetazolamide. Although there were many expected side effects, quality-of-life measures were significantly better in the acetazolamide-plus-diet group. There was no permanent morbidity from acetazolamide use.
- Positive acetazolamide-related effects on quality of life seemed to be primarily mediated by improvements in visual field, neck pain, pulsatile tinnitus, and dizziness/vertigo that outweighed the side effects of acetazolamide.
- Patients with IIH on acetazolamide as the only diuretic do not need potassium supplementation.
- Perimetry performance failures were common and were characterized by major worsening of the PMD with no change or improvement in other clinical measures.

OTHER RECENT ADVANCES IN IDIOPATHIC INTRACRANIAL HYPERTENSION

Ocular Coherence Tomography

Optical coherence tomography (OCT) is a noninvasive high-resolution (micron scale) optic nerve and retinal microstructure imaging procedure that uses light waves to take cross-section pictures by measuring backscattered or back-reflected light. There have been a variety of advances in OCT measures related to IIH over the past few years.[15,16] For example, the subsurface contour of the peripapillary retinal pigment epithelium/basement membrane junction has been shown to change with CSF pressure–lowering interventions.[17] This change can be considered a marker of structural change in IIH related to papilledema. Also, changes in the peripapillary retinal nerve fiber layer and optic nerve head volume correlate well with changes and papilledema grade. These measures provide a continuous variable rather than a categorical one and show much promise, especially for use in clinical trials. Care must be taken in individual patients though, because damage to retinal ganglion cell axons will also result in decreased optic nerve head volume.[15,16,18] These OCT methods are both sensitive to change and have excellent retest variability. In addition, the ganglion cell layer analysis may also show evidence of damage to the central 7° of the visual field, but care must be used in its interpretation because of the presence of imaging artifacts when there is moderate to severe optic disc edema present.

Choroidal wrinkles and folds are a common accompaniment to papilledema occurring in about 40% of patients with IIH. Sibony and colleagues[19] have studied choroidal folds in IIHTT subjects with both fundus photos and OCT. They identified 3 types of folds: peripapillary wrinkles occurring in 26% of photos, retinal folds in 19% of photos, and choroidal folds in 1%. Although 41% of patients have wrinkles or folds with photos, 73% have them with OCT.[19] The presence of these wrinkles and folds is an important feature in differentiating true optic disc edema from pseudopapilledema.

Medical Therapies

New findings using motivational interviewing (MI) to treat weight loss. MI is a counseling approach used to elicit behavior change that uses a collaborative patient-centered form of guiding to elicit and strengthen motivation for change. It relies on the presence of ambivalence toward the goal (by discussing and making a choice between the pros and cons of losing weight) and assists patients to actively develop their own plan to improve their health. A meta-analysis of randomized controlled trials using MI techniques to aid weight loss showed a reduction in body weight for an intervention group compared with controls of 3.24 lb.[20]

Sinclair and coworkers[21] prospectively studied intracranial pressure in women with IIH treated with a low-energy diet (a diet of foodstuffs with high volume and low calories like fresh fruits and vegetables). Twenty-five women with a body mass index (BMI) greater than 25 with IIH were treated with a 425-kcal/d diet. They found with significant reductions in weight (mean 15.7 kg), intracranial pressure decreased (mean 80 cm water, $P<.001$). Three months after the diet was discontinued, they showed no significant change in weight, and the improvement in CSF pressure was maintained.

Surgical Therapies

Case series continue to be published regarding various surgical therapies. Fonseca and colleagues[22] compared post optic nerve sheath fenestration (ONSF) visual function with post CSF shunt visual function and found a trend toward worse preoperative acuity in the ONSF cohort. Postoperative mean deviation improved by 6.35 dB in the shunted group and 6.21 dB in the ONSF group. Rizzo and coworkers reported shunting results on visual field function in 15 patients with IIH. The mean visual field mean deviation improvement was 5.63 dB. They conclude CSF shunting results in improvement in perimetry, retinal nerve fiber layer swelling, and papilledema grade in patients with IIH. Huang and colleagues[23] studied 19 shunted patients with IIH and found significant improvements in acuity but not visual field function (some of the subjects had already failed optic nerve sheath fenestration). These 3 articles are the first ones to investigate preoperative and postoperative automated visual field function in CSF shunting for IIH.

It has been known for years that CSF shunting only relieved headache in about half of the patients with IIH.[24] de Souza and colleagues[25] studied shunted patients with the diagnosis of medication overuse headache. In 180 shunted patients, 8.3% had medication overuse headaches and 12 of the 15 patients had undergone multiple shunt revisions. They concluded shunt patients should be counseled regarding medication overuse headaches.

There continue to be small uncontrolled case series of patients with IIH treated with stenting of the lateral (transverse) venous sinus; there are many apparent successes and occasional morbidity with repeat stenting occasionally needed. Subdural hematomas, subarachnoid hemorrhage, malignant cerebral edema, and prolonged anticoagulation temper the enthusiasm for this procedure. The pros and cons are discussed in a recent review.[26] Although a biologically plausible rationale for stenting selected patients with IIH with bilateral transverse sinus stenosis refractory to medical treatment exists, until there is a randomized controlled clinical trial, evidence to document efficacy, its place in the IIH treatment armamentarium remains uncertain.

A meta-analysis of 457 articles on surgical treatment of IIH yielded 30 studies with meaningful data, all with class III evidence of efficacy. A total of 332 patients were treated by ONSF, 287 by lumboperitoneal shunt (LPS), 61 by ventriculoperitoneal shunt (VPS), and 88 by dural venous sinus stenting. Visual acuity improved in 49.3%, 56.6%, 67.2%, and 84.6% of patients following VPS, LPS, ONSF, and stent placements, respectively, in these highly selected series. Shunt revision was more frequent for LPS compared with VPS. Similar improvement in visual outcomes occurred across treatment strategies. The investigators conclude there is insufficient evidence to recommend or reject any treatments modalities for IIH.[27]

Bariatric surgery has been used successfully to treat IIH for many years. Fridley and colleagues[28] reviewed the literature on the effectiveness of bariatric surgery for obese patients with IIH. They found 11 relevant publications reporting a total of 62 patients. The Roux-en-Y gastric bypass was the most common bariatric procedure used. Fifty-six (92%) of 61 patients with recorded postoperative clinical history had resolution of their presenting IIH symptoms following bariatric surgery. Thirty-four (97%) of 35 patients who had undergone preoperative and postoperative fundoscopy were found to have resolution of papilledema with the procedure. Eleven (92%) of 12 patients who had undergone preoperative and postoperative formal visual field testing had complete or nearly complete resolution of visual field deficits. In 13 patients both preoperative and postoperative CSF pressures were recorded, with an average postoperative pressure decrease of 254 mm H_2O. The investigators conclude published class IV evidence suggests that bariatric surgery may be an effective treatment of IIH in morbidly obese patients, both in terms of symptom resolution and visual outcome. The authors discuss gastric surgery in their patients with IIH with morbid obesity (BMI >40).

New Neuro-Audiologic Findings

Butros and coworkers have shown that chronically elevated CSF pressure can lead to osseous erosions, including widening of the foramen ovale and other canals and ostia. These findings may serve as a new imaging marker for IIH. But the foramen ovale can be difficult to visualize on standard MRI scans. The investigators found average foramen ovale sizes were increased in patients with IIH compared with controls, with a sensitivity of 50% and 81% specificity to detect IIH. Sensitivity and specificity of empty sella (65.9% vs 0%), posterior globe flattening (65.9% vs 4.5%), vertical tortuosity of the optic nerve (54.5% vs 9.1%), and optic nerve sheath distention (52.3% vs 11.4%) were statistically significant.[29]

Maralani and colleagues[30] also studied the accuracy of MRI in the diagnosis of IIH. In this study, 43 IIH cases and 43 controls had an MRI and magnetic resonance venogram. Partially empty sella had a sensitivity of 65.0% to detect IIH with a specificity of 95.3%; sensitivity and specificity for flattening of the posterior globes were 54% and 100% and 63% and 100% for combined stenosis score less than 4, respectively. The presence of one sign, or any combination, significantly increased the odds of a diagnosis of IIH. Their absence, however, did not rule out IIH.

Berdahl and colleagues[31] showed that BMI has a linear relationship with CSF pressure. They retrospectively studied 4235 patients undergoing lumbar puncture done at the Mayo Clinic that also had data to calculate a BMI. They found the increase in CSF pressure with increasing BMI was linear with an ($P<.001$). CSF pressure increased by 37.7% from a BMI of 18 (8.6 ± 2.1 mm Hg) to a BMI of 39 (14.1 ± 2.5 mm Hg). Unfortunately the r^2 was only 0.20, limiting the utility of correcting CSF pressure for BMI.

As discussed earlier, the transverse sinus is narrowed with increased ICP. Rohr and coworkers[32] have measured the full dural sinus tree in IIH using MRV. They studied 17 patients before and after treatment of IIH along with 7 controls. They found stenoses of the transverse sinuses resulting in cranial venous outflow obstruction in 15 of 17 (88%) of the patients with IIH. They found the obstruction normalized in 7 of 15 cases (47%) after treatment of IIH. Cranial venous outflow obstruction was not detected in the control group. Segmentation of MRV revealed decreased dural sinus volumes in general in patients with IIH compared with controls ($P = .018$). Sinus volumes increased significantly with normalization of CSF pressure, independent from resolution of transverse sinus stenoses ($P = .007$). They concluded there is a reduced volume of the venous sinus tree in IIH, which improves treatment of ICP.

REFERENCES

1. Lueck C, McIllwaine G. Interventions for idiopathic intracranial hypertension. Cochrane Database Syst Rev 2005;(3):CD003434.
2. Wall M, McDermott MP, Kieburtz KD, et al. Effect of acetazolamide on visual function in patients with idiopathic intracranial hypertension and mild visual loss: the Idiopathic Intracranial Hypertension Treatment Trial. JAMA 2014; 311(16):1641–51.
3. Corbett JJ, Savino PJ, Thompson HS, et al. Visual loss in pseudotumor cerebri. Follow-up of 57 patients from five to 41 years and a profile of 14 patients with permanent severe visual loss. Arch Neurol 1982;39:461–74.
4. Wall M, Hart WM Jr, Burde RM. Visual field defects in idiopathic intracranial hypertension (pseudotumor cerebri). Am J Ophthalmol 1983;96:654–69.
5. Lubow M, Kuhr L. Pseudotumor cerebri: comments on practical management. In: Glaser JS, Smith JL, editors. Neuro-ophthalmology, vol. IX. St Louis (MO): C.V. Mosby; 1976. p. 199–206.
6. Newborg B. Pseudotumor cerebri treated by rice reduction diet. Arch Intern Med 1974;133:802–7.
7. Gücer G, Viernstein L. Long-term intracranial pressure recording in management of pseudotumor cerebri. J Neurosurg 1978;49:256–63.
8. Friedman DI, McDermott MP, Kieburtz K, et al. The Idiopathic Intracranial Hypertension Treatment Trial: design considerations and methods. J Neuroophthalmol 2014;34(2):107–17.
9. Wall M, Kupersmith MJ, Kieburtz KD, et al. The Idiopathic Intracranial Hypertension Treatment Trial: clinical profile at baseline. JAMA Neurol 2014;71(6):693–701.
10. Wall M, Falardeau J, Fletcher WA, et al. Risk factors for poor visual outcome in patients with idiopathic intracranial hypertension. Neurology 2015;85(9):799–805.
11. Keltner JL, Johnson CA, Cello KE, et al. Baseline visual field findings in the Idiopathic Intracranial Hypertension Treatment Trial (IIHTT). Invest Ophthalmol Vis Sci 2014;55:3200–7.
12. Johnson LN, Krohel GB, Madsen RW, et al. The role of weight loss and acetazolamide in the treatment of idiopathic intracranial hypertension (pseudotumor cerebri). Ophthalmology 1998;105:2313–7.
13. Cello KE, Keltner JL, Johnson CA, et al. Factors affecting visual field outcomes in the idiopathic intracranial hypertension treatment trial. J Neuroophthalmol 2016; 36(1):6–12.
14. ten Hove MW, Friedman DI, Patel AD, et al. Safety and tolerability of acetazolamide in the idiopathic intracranial hypertension treatment trial. J Neuroophthalmol 2016; 36(1):13–9.
15. Sibony P, Kupersmith MJ, Rohlf FJ. Shape analysis of the peripapillary RPE layer in papilledema and ischemic optic neuropathy. Invest Ophthalmol Vis Sci 2011; 52:7987–95.
16. Sibony P, Kupersmith MJ, Honkanen R, et al. Effects of lowering cerebrospinal fluid pressure on the shape of the peripapillary retina in intracranial hypertension. Invest Ophthalmol Vis Sci 2014;55(12):8223–31.
17. Kupersmith MJ, Sibony P, Mandel G, et al. Optical coherence tomography of the swollen optic nerve head: deformation of the peripapillary retinal pigment epithelium layer in papilledema. Invest Ophthalmol Vis Sci 2011;52:6558–64.
18. Auinger P, Durbin M, Feldon S, et al. Baseline OCT measurements in the idiopathic intracranial hypertension treatment trial, part II: correlations and relationship to clinical features. Invest Ophthalmol Vis Sci 2014;55:8173–9.

19. Sibony PA, Kupersmith MJ, Feldon SE, et al. Retinal and choroidal folds in papilledema. Invest Ophthalmol Vis Sci 2015;56:5670–80.
20. Armstrong MJ, Mottershead TA, Ronksley PE, et al. Motivational interviewing to improve weight loss in overweight and/or obese patients: a systematic review and meta-analysis of randomized controlled trials. Obes Rev 2011;12:709–23.
21. Sinclair AJ, Burdon MA, Nightingale PG, et al. Low energy diet and intracranial pressure in women with idiopathic intracranial hypertension: prospective cohort study. BMJ 2010;341:c2701.
22. Fonseca PL, Rigamonti D, Miller NR, et al. Visual outcomes of surgical intervention for pseudotumour cerebri: optic nerve sheath fenestration versus cerebrospinal fluid diversion. Br J Ophthalmol 2014;98(10):1360–3.
23. Huang LC, Winter TW, Herro AM, et al. Ventriculoperitoneal shunt as a treatment of visual loss in idiopathic intracranial hypertension. J Neuroophthalmol 2014;34:223–8.
24. McGirt MJ, Woodworth G, Thomas G, et al. Cerebrospinal fluid shunt placement for pseudotumor cerebri-associated intractable headache: predictors of treatment response and an analysis of long-term outcomes. J Neurosurg 2004;101(4):627–32.
25. deSouza RM, Toma A, Watkins L. Medication overuse headache - an underdiagnosed problem in shunted idiopathic intracranial hypertension patients. Br J Neurosurg 2014;19:1–5.
26. Ahmed R, Friedman DI, Halmagyi GM. Stenting of the transverse sinuses in idiopathic intracranial hypertension. J Neuroophthalmol 2011;31:374–80.
27. Lai LT, Danesh-Meyer HV, Kaye AH. Visual outcomes and headache following interventions for idiopathic intracranial hypertension. J Clin Neurosci 2014;21:1670–8.
28. Fridley J, Foroozan R, Sherman V, et al. Bariatric surgery for the treatment of idiopathic intracranial hypertension. J Neurosurg 2011;114(1):34–9.
29. Butros SR, Goncalves LF, Thompson D, et al. Imaging features of idiopathic intracranial hypertension, including a new finding: widening of the foramen ovale. Acta Radiol 2012;53(6):682–8.
30. Maralani PJ, Hassanlou M, Torres C, et al. Accuracy of brain imaging in the diagnosis of idiopathic intracranial hypertension. Clin Radiol 2012;67(7):656–63.
31. Berdahl JP, Fleischman D, Zaydlarova J, et al. Body mass index has a linear relationship with cerebrospinal fluid pressure. Invest Ophthalmol Vis Sci 2012;53:1422–7.
32. Rohr A, Bindeballe J, Riedel C, et al. The entire dural sinus tree is compressed in patients with idiopathic intracranial hypertension: a longitudinal, volumetric magnetic resonance imaging study. Neuroradiology 2012;54:25–33.

Venous Sinus Stenting for Idiopathic Intracranial Hypertension: Where Are We Now?

Marc J. Dinkin, MD[a,b,c,*], Athos Patsalides, MD, MPH[d]

KEYWORDS

• Idiopathic intracranial hypertension • Venous sinus stenosis • Stenting
• Papilledema • Visual fields • Magnetic resonance venography • Angiography

KEY POINTS

- An increasing amount of evidence suggests that stenosis at the junction of the transverse and sigmoid sinuses contributes to increased intracranial pressure in idiopathic intracranial hypertension.
- Stenting of the stenosis in medically refractory, medically intolerant, or fulminant patients seems to result in improvement in symptoms, papilledema, and intracranial pressure in most patients assessed.
- Prospective, controlled trials comparing venous stenting with alternative surgical therapies or maximal medical therapy are needed to better assess the efficacy of venous sinus stenting.

Video content accompanies this article at http://www.neurologic.theclinics.com.

INTRODUCTION

Idiopathic intracranial hypertension (IIH) is a condition that causes increased intracranial hypertension, typically in obese women of childbearing age, in the absence of

Conflicts of Interest: No conflicting relationship exists for any author of this study.
Financial Support: None.
[a] Department of Ophthalmology, New York Presbyterian Hospital, Weill Cornell Medical College, New York, NY, USA; [b] Department of Neurology, New York Presbyterian Hospital, Weill Cornell Medical College, New York, NY, USA; [c] Department of Neurosurgery, New York Presbyterian Hospital, Weill Cornell Medical College, New York, NY, USA; [d] Division of Interventional Neuroradiology, Department of Neurological Surgery, New York Presbyterian Hospital, Weill Cornell Medical College, 525 E 68th Street, New York, NY 10065, USA
* Corresponding author. Department of Ophthalmology, New York Presbyterian Hospital, Weill Cornell Medical College, 1305 York Avenue, 11th Floor, New York, NY 10065.
E-mail address: mjd2004@med.cornell.edu

Neurol Clin 35 (2017) 59–81
http://dx.doi.org/10.1016/j.ncl.2016.08.006
neurologic.theclinics.com

mass lesion, venous thrombosis, or meningitic process. Although first described as a meningitis serosa by Quincke[1] in 1893, it was later called pseudotumor cerebri, then benign intracranial hypertension, and then, in recognition of its unclear cause, IIH. Symptoms typically include positional headache; horizontal diplopia from abducens palsies; pulse synchronous tinnitus (PST); and, most significantly, visual field loss and transient visual obscurations (TVOs) from papilledema. Although papilledema typically resolves with treatment of the disease, prolonged or severe disc edema may leave up to 25% of patients with visual field loss,[2] and, in more severe cases, even visual acuity may be permanently affected.

In Walter Dandy's[3] seminal article on the disorder, in which he laid out criteria, including increased intracranial pressure (ICP) without mass, and with normal contents on spinal fluid examination, he pondered the possible causes of increased ICP in these patients:

> *We may well be dealing with a condition that has more than one underlying anatomic or etiologic basis.*

Although the dynamics of cerebrospinal fluid (CSF) flow are likely to play a role in IIH, it is interesting that Dandy[3] entertained a vascular contribution as well:

> *The only other possible explanation of the increased intracranial pressure is by variance in the intracranial bed probably by vasomotor control.*

Dandy's[3] recognition of the importance of hemodynamics in ICP foretold an interest in venous hemodynamics and its role in IIH that has emerged over the last 2 decades.

Although some CSF drains through lymphatics and from spinal roots,[4] a primary means of CSF outflow is through the arachnoid granulations and into the cortical venous sinuses. Thus, venous sinus thrombosis or occlusion by an adjacent tumor may mimic IIH and cause significant vision loss from papilledema. Many practitioners therefore include magnetic resonance venography (MRV) in the work-up of IIH, although this practice remains controversial.[5] However, it has become clear over the last 2 decades that most patients with IIH harbor stenosis at the junction of the transverse sinus (TS) and sigmoid sinus (SS) on 1 or both sides,[6] leading to the hypothesis that this stenosis might be playing a role in the increase of ICP. In 1995, King and colleagues[7] showed an increase in venous sinus pressure in the superior sagittal sinus and proximal TS of 7 patients with IIH, with a mean pressure gradient along the TS of 13.3 mm Hg, (vs a mean of 1.4 mm Hg in controls), suggesting that stenoses could affect venous flow and therefore CSF dynamics. In 2 patients with minocycline-induced IIH, there was no observed gradient, suggesting that the gradient played a role in truly idiopathic IIH as opposed to secondary IIH induced by a medication.

Although IIH is typically treated with acetazolamide, which has been shown to be more effective than diet alone in mild IIH in the Idiopathic Intracranial Hypertension Treatment Trial (IIHTT),[8] the condition can be resistant to the medication in up to 10% of patients,[9] requiring a surgical therapy such as optic nerve sheath fenestration or ventriculoperitoneal shunt (VPS) or lumboperitoneal shunt (LPS). Up to 2.9% of patients present with a fulminant picture with central visual field and significant acuity loss[10] and cannot wait for acetazolamide to take effect, also requiring the quick fix of a surgical procedure. Although fenestration and shunts have a long record of efficacy in IIH, they both carry certain risks of complication, including diplopia and rare traumatic vision loss in fenestration[11] and overdrainage and infection with shunts.[12] It was therefore not long before groups began attempting to treat IIH with stenting of venous sinus stenosis (VSS) in the hope that this would reverse the gradient observed in King and colleagues'[7] study and therefore the increase in ICP.[13] The first study by Higgins and colleagues[14] included 12 patients, 5 of whom had failed a prior shunt, although only 3 underwent prestent lumbar puncture (LP), and only 8 of them had papilledema before treatment. The results were mixed, with only 4 patients showing resolution of papilledema, and 7 out of 12 showing resolution of improvement in headache, and there were serious complications, including in-stent thrombosis in 2 patients, but their work prepared the way for numerous case reports[15–24] and future studies.[25–33] The largest study included 52 patients, and reported resolution of papilledema in all 46 patients who had it before stenting.[34]

To date, including numerous case reports, the authors were able to identify in the literature a total of 282 patients who have undergone venous stent placement for IIH. This article discusses the potential pathophysiology of VSS in IIH in greater detail, and summarizes the results of the available studies to date, also discussing future directions that might be taken to better understand the role of stenting in this disease.

HYPOTHETICAL ROLE OF VENOUS SINUS STENOSIS IN IDIOPATHIC INTRACRANIAL HYPERTENSION

Critics of the role of VSS in IIH have proposed that VSS might be the consequence and not the cause of intracranial hypertension. King[35] showed an amelioration of venous hypertension in 8 patients with IIH following CSF removal during venous manometry, whereas Rohr and colleagues[36] showed a reversal of VSS following CSF diversion procedures in 3 patients, and argued that patients with VSS should not undergo stenting if a CSF diversion procedure showed such reversibility. Bono and colleagues[37] showed the opposite phenomenon in 9 patients whose VSS persisted after medical therapy for IIH. So is VSS the consequence of intracranial hypertension or the cause?

There are a minority of cases in which VSS seems to be the consequence of fixed anatomic variations, such as a septal band, swollen arachnoid granulation, chronic thrombosis, or trabecula, and thus might be a primary factor leading to IIH, but even in these intrinsic cases, a "second hit" must have occurred (additional risk factors such as weight gain or change in CSF production) and, in conjunction with the presumably long-standing stenosis, led to high ICP. In some case, the intrinsic stenosis seems to be congenital, supported by a study that showed a narrowing or absence of the perisinus bony groove in 5 out of 23 and 8 out of 23 cases of IIH-associated VSS respectively.[38] Kelly and colleagues[39] found bilateral VSS in 7 patients, none of whom had papilledema or symptoms of increased ICP, suggesting a presymptomatic version of VSS and supporting the notion that intrinsic VSS may require a second hit before intracranial hypertension ensues.

However, in most patients with IIH VSS seems to be extrinsic; that is, it is a consequence of increased ICP, and therefore reversible with a reduction in ICP. Should Rohr and colleagues'[36] advice therefore be followed, with consideration of stenting reserved only for those intrinsic cases?

Clinicians who would consider stenting for extrinsic stenosis put forth the positive feedback loop argument that some unknown factor leads to a mild increase in ICP, perhaps not enough to cause major symptoms but sufficient to cause extrinsic VSS. The stenosis in turn leads to higher ICP, which leads to greater stenosis, and, by way of this vicious cycle, the ICP reaches levels that produce papilledema and vision loss (Video 1). This approach has been modeled as a Starling-like resistor,[40] which is a fluid-filled collapsible tube that sits in an air-filled chamber whose pressure can be modulated to collapse the tube, thus increasing the resistance to flow. In the case of VSS, the equivalent of the air in the chamber (ie, ICP) is increased when flow is reduced, creating an unstable system (**Fig. 1**). By placing a stent in the sinus, the

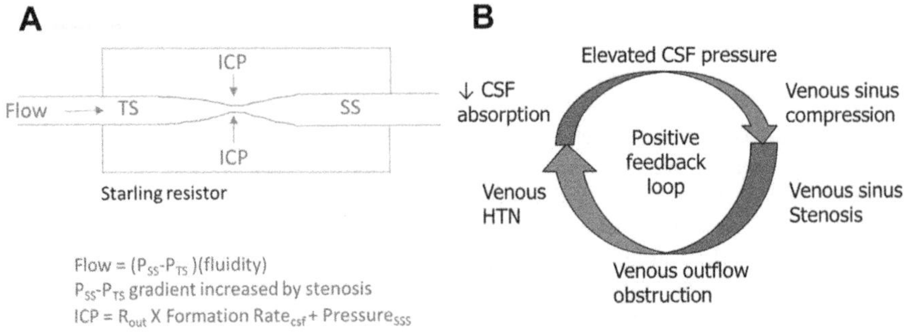

Fig. 1. (*A*) Flow through the stenotic segment of the TS-SS may be modeled as a Starling resistor, whereby it is proportionate to the difference between the distal (SS) and proximal (TS) segment pressures (trans-stenotic gradient). This flow in turn affects outflow resistance to CSF, which increases ICP, causing greater stenosis and therefore an even greater trans-stenotic gradient. This positive feedback loop is illustrated in (*B*). CSF, cerebrospinal fluid; HTN, hypertension; ICP, intracranial pressure; PSS, pressure at the sigmoid sinus; PTS, pressure at the transverse sinus; Rout, resistance to outflow from of CSF; SS, sigmoid sinus; TS, transverse sinus; Venous HTN, venous hypertension.

tube is no longer collapsible, the system becomes stable, and theoretically the ICP can return to the only slightly increased level at which it had been before the positive loop began (**Fig. 2**). Although this theory may support stenting of extrinsic VSS, the authors note that, in our study of 13 patients with medically refractory IIH, the greatest reduction in ICP after stenting occurred in 4 of the 5 patients whose stenosis was thought to be intrinsic at presentation, suggesting that the effect of stenting may be greater in those cases with a fixed anatomic VSS.[33]

EVIDENCE FOR VENOUS STENTING: A META-ANALYSIS

Having reviewed the theoretic role of VSS in IIH and the rationale for therapeutic stenting, this article now considers the available data in the literature to date to evaluate the safety and efficacy of venous stenting. Using PubMed, the authors searched for literature regarding venous sinus stenting for IIH and found 16 reported studies (15 retrospective and 1 prospective) with 3 or more patients, and 9 single case reports, totaling 282 patients. Mean clinical follow-up after stenting was 21.2 months (follow-up duration by study is shown in **Fig. 3**). When researchers from 1 group published more than once covering the same patients, we included the larger study, to avoid counting patients more than once. We combined data from these available articles and performed a meta-analysis of patient demographics, stent characteristics, and subjective and objective outcomes. The median number of subjects in the studies was 17 (range, 3–52). One study[41] included 24 subjects, but 8 of them underwent only angioplasty, whereas the remaining 16 underwent stenting. Because the results for the two groups were combined, the 8 patients who only underwent angioplasty could not be separated out from the 282. For means reported, values were weighted according to the number of patients per study.

Previous Surgeries

Of the 282 patients, 27 (9.6%) had been previously treated with optic nerve sheath fenestration (ONSF), whereas 24 (8.5%) had previously received a shunt that had failed. None had undergone bariatric surgery or cranial expansion surgery.

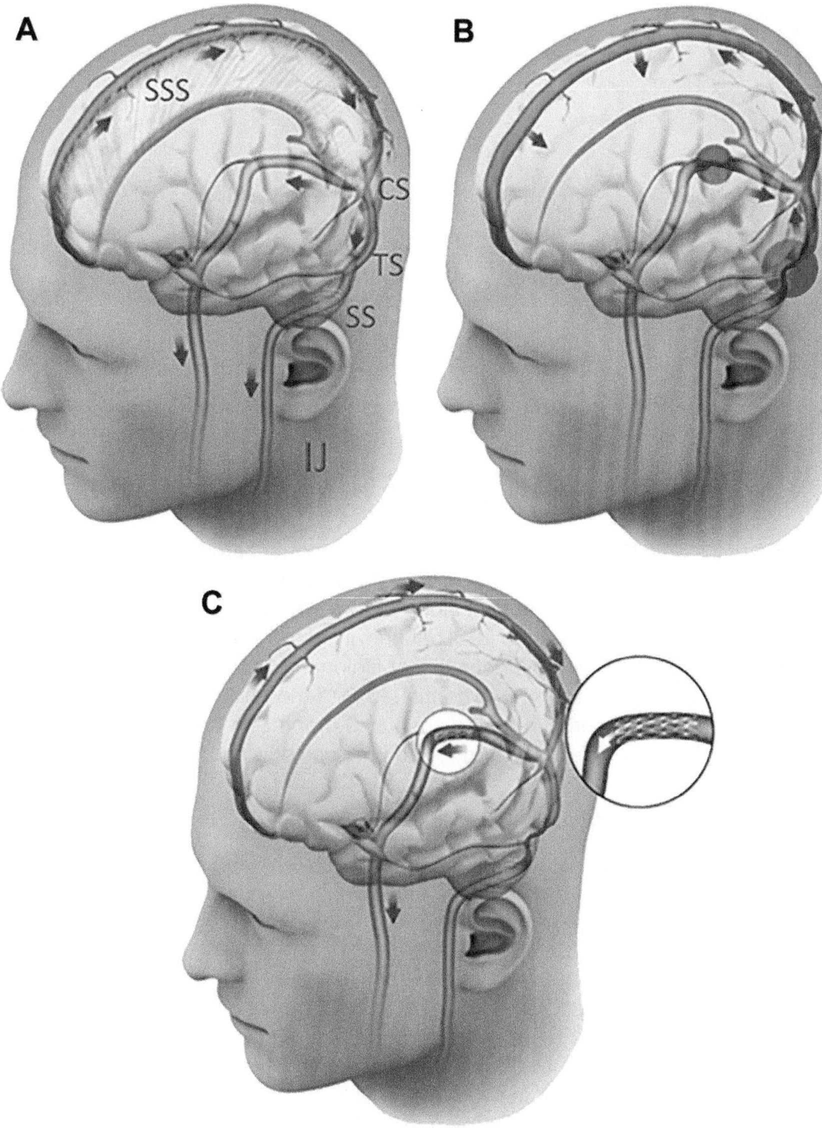

Fig. 2. (*A*) Normal sinus anatomy shows flow of CSF into the sagittal sinus (SSS), from which venous blood flows to the confluence of sinuses (CS) through the TS and SS to the internal jugular veins (IJ). (*B*) Stenosis at the TS-SS junction (*red circles*) obstructs venous outflow, leading to higher pressure proximal to the stenoses. (*C*) Stenting of the region of stenosis restores normal outflow and pressures.

Antiplatelet Therapy and Anticoagulation

There has been considerable variation in the type and duration of antiplatelet therapy used before and after VSS. Higgins and colleagues[13,14] placed their patients on lifelong aspirin and on 2 months of warfarin. However, in their early cases they did not start antiplatelet therapy before stenting, a practice to which they attribute the

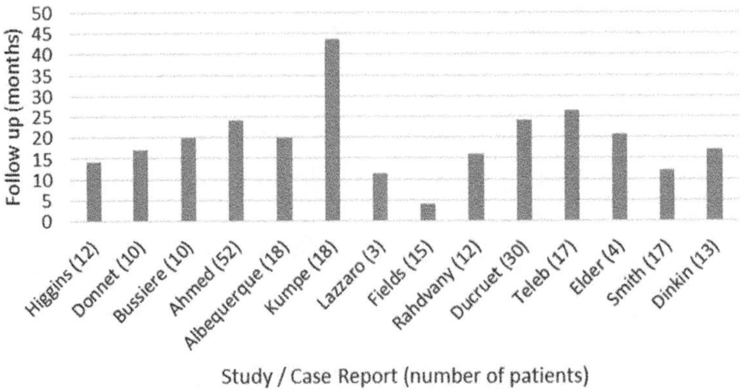

Fig. 3. Mean clinical follow-up by study. Mean across all patients was 21.2 months. Note a mean follow-up time of 43.7 months in Kumpe, in which the maximum follow-up period was 136 months.

occurrence of in-stent thrombosis in 2 patients. Subsequent studies ranged from just 3 months of clopidogrel[25] to lifelong clopidogrel and aspirin.[42] Out of 16 studies, clopidogrel alone was used in 1, aspirin alone in 1 and both in 14. In addition, warfarin was used in the perioperative period in all patients in 1 study[14] and in select patients in 1 study.[26] Aspirin was continued indefinitely or lifelong in 6 studies and for as little as 6 months in 5 studies. Clopidogrel was continued for 1 month in 1 study, 3 months in 4 studies, greater than 3 months in 2 studies, 3 to 6 months in 1 study, 6 months in 4 studies, 6 to 12 months in 1 study, and for an unspecified period in 1 study.

Features of Stenosis and Trans-stenotic Gradient

Detailed data regarding stenosis and stenting were found in 241 patients in the literature. The type of stenosis was described as intrinsic in 50 patients, extrinsic in 31 patients, and combined intrinsic and extrinsic in 32 patients. For the rest of the patients the type of stenosis was not specified. The degree of stenosis has only been reported in a few studies[33,42,43] and averaged 63.7%. The length of stenosis was only described in 1 study, and was 22.7 mm.[33] The side of stenting (in the subset in which it was reported) was right in 119 patients, left in 53 patients, and bilateral in 9 patients. The right-left discrepancy probably results from the right sinus more often being dominant, in which case its stenosis is clinically important. Location of stent placement, when reported, was in the TS/SS junction (n = 96), the TS (85), internal jugular vein (2) and SS (1). In 5 patients, placement in the TS was reported, but review of the images was most consistent with TS/SS junction. A reduction in trans-stenotic gradient (TSG) was reported in most patients who underwent poststent venography, although some studies did not report poststent TSG. The mean TSG reduced from 20.4 mm Hg to 2.4 mm Hg following stenting.

The relevance of the various properties of the stenosis to the patients' clinical course remains to be elucidated. A study of 46 patients with VSS in 1 institution showed a median average stenosis of 56% and showed no correlation between the degree or location of the stenosis with clinical course, visual field grade, or CSF pressure.[44,45] Furthermore, Kumpe, in a response to a letter from Ahmed and colleagues,[46] reported that the 5 patients in their group who developed hemodynamic deterioration requiring a second stent did not have higher venous pressures at presentation, or a higher TSG, than those patients who did not require a second stent. However, they did note that deterioration only occurred in patients with extrinsic stenosis, sparing those with intrinsic only. It is suggested that, when extrinsic stenosis is blocked along one segment, a second compressible segment is more likely to compensate in the future. However, when an intrinsic stenosis is stented, a secondary deterioration is less likely, because this stenosis is ostensibly the primary cause of the increased ICP. In our study, the mean improvement in opening pressure (OP) in the intrinsic group (30.2 cm H_2O) was greater than that of the extrinsic group (14.75 cm H_2O).[33] The authors postulate that a greater effect on ICP with stenting of intrinsic stenosis reflects a more fundamental role of these stenoses on the pathophysiology of IIH than extrinsic stenoses (**Table 1**).

Effect on Intracranial Pressure

Of the 282 patients in the literature, 213 underwent an LP before stenting but only 74 underwent a follow-up LP to directly assess the effect of stenting on the ICP. Prestent mean OP (among the 170 patients in whom values were reported) was 36.05 cm H_2O.

Within the group in which prestent and poststent OPs were reported ($n = 69$), the mean ICP reduced from 36.4 to 20.4 cm H_2O. ICP seems to have been reduced in all but 1 patient,[33] who was found to have new stenosis adjacent to the stent 1 week before the planned LP. In this case, the OP did reduce following placement of a second stent. **Fig. 4** shows the OPs before and after stenting as calculated for each study.

Effect on Symptoms

Sorting out the prevalence of symptoms at presentation and the percentage that improved after stenting was difficult, because, in many of studies, patients were simply stated to have visual symptoms, which could include TVO, diplopia, blurry vision, or recognition of field defects. In some studies, "symptoms" were said to improve after stenting, but it is not clear what these symptoms were.

Out of 282 patients, 260 (92.2%) presented with headache, 84 (32.3%) of whom experienced resolution and 131 (50.4%) experienced improvement. With 17% experiencing no improvement and more than 67% still experiencing headaches to some degree, the success rate of venous stenting for headache is imperfect but compares favorably with that of other procedures. In Lai and colleagues' comparison of ONSF, shunting, and stenting, headache improved in 36.5% of ONSF patients, 62.5% of VPS patients, 75.2% of LPS patients, and 82.9% of those treated with stenting.[47] No matter the procedure, it seems that improvement in headache is a poor marker for improvement in ICP because papilledema resolved in many patients with ongoing headache. Causes for refractory headache include failure to reduce ICP, migraine, tension headaches, and medication rebound headaches.

Sixty-two (22.0%) of the 282 stented patients experienced TVO, 47 (75.8%) of whom experienced complete resolution, which, as expected, is similar to the percentage of patients who experienced improvement or resolution of papilledema. Of the 94 patients (33.3%) with PST, 81 (86.2%) experienced complete resolution. In our experience, this symptom resolved in all patients immediately after stenting, reflecting the recognition that the stenosis produces this symptom. A series of 46 patients with PST was reported in which only 3 had intracranial hypertension, suggesting that VSS can cause PST without concomitant intracranial hypertension. In that series, all patients experienced immediate resolution after stenting.

Diplopia (typically from abducens palsies) was present in 36 (12.8%) of the patients at presentation and resolved in 33 (91.7%) after stenting. Many studies did not

Table 1
Features of stenosis, stent placement and trans-stenotic gradient among 237 patients with idiopathic intracranial hypertension

		Stenosis					TSG (mm Hg)			Side			Stent		
Authors	n	Mean (%)	Mean length (mm)	Intrinsic	Extrinsic	Both	Cutoff to Stent	Mean Before	Mean After	Right	Left	B/L	Type	Stents/ Patients	Location
Higgins et al,[14] 2003	12	NA	NA	NA	—	—	NA	18.9	5.9	0	0	2	NA	14/12	NA
Ogungbo et al,[15] 2003	1	NA	NA	NA	—	—	NA	25	NA	1	0	0	SE	1	TS/SS
Rajpal et al,[16] 2005	1	NA	NA	NA	—	—	NA	18.4	NA	1	0	0	SE	1	TS
Paquet et al,[17] 2008	1	NA	NA	NA	—	—	NA	15	NA	1	0	0	NA	1	TS
Crosa et al,[18] 2007	1	NA	NA	NA	—	—	NA	16	NA	0	1	0	SE	1	SS
Donnet et al,[25] 2008	10	NA	NA	6	4	0	NA	19.1	NA	7	2	1	SE	1	NA
Arac et al,[19] 2009	1	NA	NA	NA	—	—	NA	13	2	1	0	0	SE	1	TS
Bussière et al,[26] 2010	10	NA	NA	NA	—	—	10	24.6	11.2 (n = 8)	8	2	0	SE, BE	1	TS = 10
Zheng et al,[20] 2010	1	NA	NA	1	0	0	NA	11.7	0	0	1	0	SE	1	TS
Crawford & McGrath,[21] 2010	1	NA	NA	NA	—	—	NA	25	1	0	1	0	SE	1	TS
Spilberg et al,[22] 2010	1	NA	NA	1	0	0	NA	23	NA	0	1	0	SE	1	TS

Ahmed et al,[34] 2011	52	NA	NA	17	11	24	8	19.07	0.65 (n = 50)	36	16	2	SA, BA	72/52	TS = 52
Kumpe et al,[28] 2012	18	NA	NA	11	3	4	NA	21.5	2.5	12	7	0	SA, BA	19/18	TS/SS = 18
Ahmed et al,[46] 2012	18	NA	NA	9	5	4	7	20	0	NA	NA	NA	SA, BA	19/18	TS
Lazzaro et al,[42] 2012	3	83.3	NA	NA	—	—	NA	32	0.3	1	2	0	SA, BA	1	TS/SS = 3
Fields et al,[29] 2013	15	NA	NA	NA	—	—	10	24	4	9	2	2	SA	19/15	TS/SS = 10, TS = 5
Radvany et al,[30] 2013	12	NA	NA	NA	—	—	4	12.4	1.25	10	2	0	NA	14/12	TS = 12
Fargen et al,[23] 2013	1	NA	NA	NA	—	—	NA	55	NA	1	0	0	SA	1	TS/SS
Ding et al,[24] 2014	1	NA	NA	NA	—	—	NA	20	3	0	1	0	SA	1	TS
Ducruet et al,[43] 2014	30	>50%	NA	NA	—	—	10	21.4	NA	10	8	NA	SA	36/30	TS/SS = 18, IJV = 1
Teleb et al,[31] 2015	17	NA	NA	NA	—	—	NA	13.7	1.7	11	4	2	SA, BA	25/18	TS/SS = 15, TS = 4, IJV = 1
Smith et al,[32] 2016	17	NA	NA	NA	—	—	15	26.06	1.18	NA	—	NA	SA	19/17	TS/SS = 17
Dinkin & Patsalides,[33] 2016	13	81.5	22.7	5	8	0	8	21.3	3.2	10	3	0	SA	14/13	TS/SS = 13
Total	237			50	31	32				119	53	7			
Mean (weighted)		63.70%					9.0	20.4	2.4						

Abbreviations: B/L, bilateral; BE, balloon expandable; TSG, trans-stenotic gradient; SE, self-expandable.

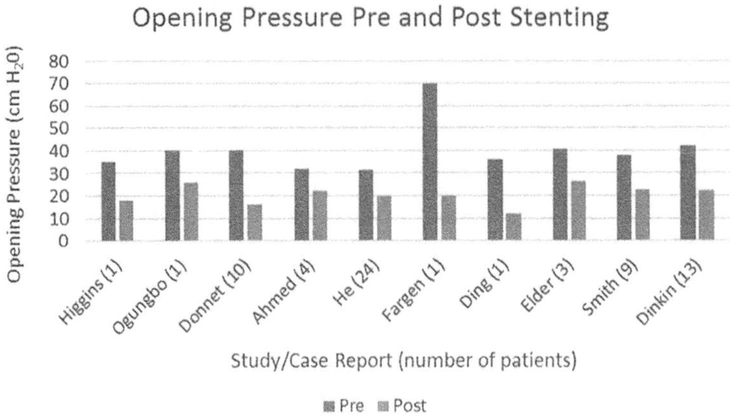

Fig. 4. Mean OPs by study, before and after venous stenting among 68 patients who underwent LP both before and after the procedure.

differentiate between diplopia, blurry vision, and TVO, but instead reported visual symptoms, which improved or resolved in 78 of 89 patients (87.6%). **Table 2** summarizes clinical symptoms before and after stenting.

Effect on Papilledema

Out of 282 patients, only 199 (70.6%) presented with papilledema (Albuquerque and colleagues[27] reported that patients presented with either papilledema *or* high ICP), indicating that stenting was not always reserved for patients with an active threat to vision. Of these, 145 patients (72.9%) experienced resolution, 24 (12%) improved, and 15 (7.5%) were reported as resolved or improved. Only 16 (8% of those with papilledema at onset) were left with optic atrophy, suggesting that the speed of ICP normalization following stenting is generally sufficient to prevent irreversible optic nerve damage.

Visual Outcomes

Visual acuity

A minority of studies offered quantitative data regarding visual acuity. Including case reports, some degree of visual acuity loss was reported in 166 out of 282 (58.9%) patients, with improvement or stabilization reported in 97 out of 166 (58.4% of eyes with acuity loss). Of the 166, 149 (89.8%) had greater than or equal to 20/25 visual acuity after stenting. Seven studies with a total of 78 patients provided quantitative visual acuity information either per eye or as a mean of the right and left eye and 6 of those studies provided prestent acuities as well. The time of poststent assessment was at last follow-up in 1 series[25] and varied between 3 and 12 months (mean, 8.9 months). The authors of this review calculated the OU acuity (the average of the right and left eye acuity) for each patient in these studies, before and after stenting. The mean prestent OU acuity was LogMAR 0.226 (Snellen 20/34) and the mean poststent OU acuity was LogMAR 0.115 (Snellen 20/28).

Visual fields

Quantitative data on visual fields were found in 3 studies.[30,33,34] Among 154 eyes in these 3 studies, some degree of initial visual field loss was observed in 107, with an improvement occurring in 80 and a worsening in 9. Quantitative analysis of mean deviation (MD) scores was reported in 2 studies for a total of 37 eyes. The average MD at onset was −9.05 dB and improved to −5.58 dB. The mean change in MD was +3.47 dB (range, −11.73 to +28.08 dB). Because the primary cause of disability in patients with IIH is visual field loss, it is imperative that future studies include visual field data, preferably including quantitative analysis of MD. **Table 3** summarizes visual assessment before and after stenting.

Optical Coherence Tomography Data

Spectral domain (SD) optical coherence tomography (OCT) uses low-coherence light to evaluate the thickness of individual retina layers, including that of the retinal nerve fiber layer (RNFL), which becomes edematous in the setting of active papilledema.[48] As such, SD-OCT allows a quantified assessment of papilledema before and after a given procedure, including venous sinus stenting. To date, 3 studies have reported SD-OCT data in patients undergoing venous stenting. The first studied the mean RNFL (mRNFL) once before stenting and then on 3 occasions after stenting (before 1 month, between 1 and3 months, and once after 3 months).[49] The mRNFL normalized (reaching ≤108 μm) in 8 out of 10 patients by the last SD-OCT, which was performed at 3 months in the 2 patients who did not normalize. One eye of a patient who was followed for 26 months also did not normalize (reaching 116 μm). Most eyes normalized around 80 days and the improvement followed a linear regression model. The second study showed a reduction in mRNFL in 8 out of 11 patients who underwent OCT, even though 2 of them did not have clinical papilledema at presentation, and the remaining 3 patients maintained their initial normal mean thicknesses.[32] Specific values for mRNFL were not reported but, in the 3 patients whose RNFL was normal at onset and remained stable, there was improvement in visual acuity, suggesting an alternative cause of the initial acuity loss not captured by mRNFL thickness. The third study prospectively performed OCT on 23 eyes of 12 patients at 3 months after stenting, and found a reduction in the average mRNFL from 205.4 μm to 89.1 μm, with maintenance of normal thickness in 2 eyes.[33] Normalization of mRNFL occurred in 12 out of 14 eyes with increased thickness at presentation and in the remaining 2 eyes (of 1 patient) in the subsequent months. Combining the 3 studies, there was improvement in mRNFL in 24 out of 26 patients following venous stenting. However, although assessment of mRNFL allows a quantitative evaluation of papilledema, it has several limitations, most notably that a normal mRNFL may reflect a combination of thickening and atrophy, and can therefore be falsely reassuring. As such, OCT data for venous stenting must always be assessed in the context of clinical and visual outcomes.

Adverse Events

The most common adverse event was a headache ipsilateral to the stent, typically lasting for only a few days, reflective of dural stretch by the stent. Some studies reported this frequency qualitatively ("usually" or "in most"), but, assuming a prevalence in 75% of the patients in those studies, this complication was observed in 84 out of 278 patients (30.2%). This finding is likely an underestimate because studies that did not mention it may have grouped it with persistent IIH headaches. In-stent thrombosis occurred in 2 of the first patients in the first trial,[14] and was attributed by the investigators to their early practice of not starting antiplatelet therapy until after stenting. A total of 4 intracranial bleeds occurred (1.4%) and deserve discussion.[28,34,41] Kumpe and colleagues[28] described stasis of flow during stent placement with secondary subdural hematoma (SDH) and subarachnoid hemorrhage (SAH), which left a residual mild foot weakness, but this was in the setting of a

Table 2
Symptoms before and after venous stenting among 282 patients with idiopathic intracranial hypertension

		Headache Outcome			TVO		Pulsatile Tinnitus		Diplopia		Visual symptoms	
	n	Before	Resolved	Improved	Before	After	Before	After	Before	After	Before	Improved/Resolved
Higgins et al,[14] 2003	12	12	5	2	4	0	0	0	0	0	NA	NA
Ogungbo et al,[15] 2003	1	1	1	0	1	0	0	0	0	0	1	1
Rajpal et al,[16] 2005	1	1	1	0	0	0	0	0	1	0	1	1
Paquet et al,[17] 2008	1	1	0	1	0	0	0	0	0	0	0	0
Crosa et al,[18] 2007	1	1	0	1	0	0	0	0	0	0	1	1
Donnet et al,[25] 2008	10	10	6	2	10	0	9	0	0	0	10	5
Arac et al,[19] 2009	1	1	0	1	1	NA	1	0	0	0	0	0
Bussière et al,[26] 2010	10	10	2	8	0	0	3	NA	0	0	NA	NA
Zheng et al,[20] 2010	1	1	1	0	0	0	0	0	0	0	1	1
Spilberg et al,[22] 2010	1	1	1	0	0	0	0	0	0	0	1	1
Ahmed et al,[34] 2011	52	43	35	8	19	0	17	0	6	0	25	25
Albuquerque et al,[27] 2011	18	15	2	12	NA	NA	NA	NA	NA	NA	NA	NA
Kumpe et al,[28] 2012	18	12	2	8	NA	NA	NA	NA	NA	NA	NA	NA
Ahmed et al,[46] 2012	18	17	0	16	0	0	11	0	0	0	NA	NA
He et al,[41] 2012	24	24	10	6	NA	NA	2	NA	6	NA	NA	NA

Lazzaro et al,[42] 2012	3	3	0	2	0	NA	0	NA	0	NA	1	1
Fields et al,[29] 2013	15	15	2	8	0	NA	14	3	0	NA	NA	NA
Radvany et al,[30] 2013	12	12	2	5	NA	NA	11	3	NA	NA	NA	NA
Fargen et al,[23] 2013	1	1	NA	NA	NA	NA	NA	NA	NA	NA	NA	NA
Ding et al,[24] 2014	1	1	1	0	NA	NA	NA	NA	NA	NA	NA	NA
Ducruet et al,[43] 2014	30	27	0	19	NA	NA	NA	NA	NA	NA	NA	NA
Teleb et al,[31] 2015	17	17	9	6	NA	NA	5	1	NA	NA	18	14
Elder 2015	4	4	0	4	0	0	2	1	0	0	NA	NA
Smith et al,[32] 2016	17	17	0	15	17	13	8	5	17	NA	17	15
Dinkin & Patsalides,[33] 2016	13	13	4	7	10	2	11	0	6	3	13	13
Total	282	260	84	131	62	15	94	13	36	3	89	78
Percentage	—	92.2	32.3	50.4	22.0	24.2	33.3	13.8	12.8	8.3	31.6	87.6

For columns headed Before, percentage refers to the percentage of the total group of 282 who presented with that symptom. For columns headed After, Improved, or Resolved, percentage refers to the percentage of patients who presented with the symptom who still had the symptom (After), who experienced resolution (Resolved), or improvement (Improved).

Table 3
Neuro-ophthalmic assessment before and after stenting among 282 patients with idiopathic intracranial hypertension

		Visual Acuity (Eyes)			Visual Fields (Eyes)				Papilledema (Patients)			
	n	Initial loss	Improved	Final Acuity ≥20/25	Loss Initial	↑	No Δ	↓	Present at Onset	Resolved	↑	Optic Atrophy
Higgins et al,[14] 2003	12	NA	NA	NA	NA	NA	NA	NA	8	4	1	0
Ogungbo et al,[15] 2003	1	NA	NA	NA	NA	NA	NA	NA	1	0	1	0
Rajpal et al,[16] 2005	1	2	NA	NA	NA	NA	NA	NA	1	1	0	0
Paquet et al,[17] 2008	1	2	2	2	NA	NA	NA	NA	1	1	0	0
Crosa et al,[18] 2007	1	2	NA	NA	NA	NA	NA	NA	1	0	1	0
Donnet et al,[25] 2008	10	15	12	13	NA	NA	NA	NA	10	10	0	2
Arac et al,[19] 2009	1	2	NA	NA	NA	NA	NA	NA	0	0	0	0
Bussière et al,[26] 2010	10	8	5	15	NA	NA	NA	NA	9	5	4	1
Zheng et al,[20] 2010	1	NA	NA	NA	NA	NA	NA	NA	1	1	0	0
Spilberg et al,[22] 2010	1	NA	NA	NA	NA	NA	NA	NA	1	1	0	0
Ahmed et al,[34] 2011	52	26	18	48	60[b]	46	14	0	46	46	0	4
Albuquerque et al,[27] 2011	18	NA	NA	NA	NA	NA	NA	NA	NA[c]	NA	NA	NA
Kumpe et al,[28] 2012	18	NA	30[a]	NA	NA	NA	NA	NA	17	15	0	0
Ahmed et al,[46] 2012	18	3	1	NA	7	5	2	1	13	13	0	1

He et al,[41] 2012	24	36	26	NA	NA	NA	NA	NA	14	5	5	1
Lazzaro et al,[42] 2012	3	4	4	NA	NA	2	1	NA	3	1	2	1
Fields et al,[29] 2013	15	28	10	20	NA	NA	NA	NA	15	15	0	1
Radvany et al,[30] 2013	12	24	12	22	21	12	7	5	12	11	0	0
Fargen et al,[23] 2013	1	2	0	0	NA	NA	NA	NA	1	1	0	2
Ding et al,[24] 2014	1	NA	NA	NA	1	1	0	0	1	NA	NA	NA
Ducruet et al,[43] 2014	30	NA	NA	NA	NA	NA	NA	NA	NA	NA	NA	NA
Teleb et al,[31] 2015	17	NA	NA	NA	NA	NA	NA	NA	16	0	15[d]	NA
Elder 2015	4	6	2	6	6	4	0	2	4	4	0	1
Smith et al,[32] 2016	17	NA	NA	NA	NA	NA	NA	NA	11	0	9	NA
Dinkin & Patsalides,[33] 2016	13	6	5	23	25	19	3	2	13	11	1	2
Total	282	166	97	149	120	89	27	10	199	145	39	16
Percentage	—	58.9	58.4	89.8	42.6	74.2	22.5	8.3	70.6	72.9	19.6	8.0

Symbols: ↑, improved; ↓, worsened; Δ, change.

[a] Improved or stabilized.

[b] Estimated based on data reported as numbers of patients.

[c] Presented with either high ICP or papilledema.

[d] Either resolved or improved.

parasagittal arteriovenous malformation and secondary contralateral sinus thrombosis, so it is difficult to characterize this patient's intracranial hypertension as truly idiopathic. Ahmed and colleagues[34] reported 2 intracranial hemorrhages: an SDH after guidewire perforation and an unexplained SDH/SAH contralateral to the side of stent placement, but both patients recovered fully. Other serious complications include stent migration, contrast extravasation, and anaphylaxis, all occurring in 1 patient each (0.41%), and transient hearing loss in 4 patients (1.6%). The mechanism for transient hearing loss is unknown, but may involve a temporary, stent-related disturbance in the outflow of the cochlear veins, which in some patients drain directly into the TS (although most drain into the petrosal sinus). Such outflow might cause hearing loss by way of cochlear ischemia or increased inner ear pressure, as it seems to do in some cases of venous sinus thrombosis.[50] Note that there was 1 death reported in which uncontrolled cerebral edema was attributed to hypercapnia in the setting of ventilation under general anesthesia.[51] Given the low risk of death from general anesthesia (<4 per 1 million),[52] it is hard to fully rule out some contribution to the cerebral edema by venous stasis related to the stent. Levitt and colleagues[53] investigated this and found no immediate effect on venous outflow from the vein of Labbe even though the stent spanned the venous ostium of the vein in 92.1% of their patients, but our group has noted stasis in a cortical vein at the time of stenting in 2 patients, prompting treatment with heparin for a few days to prevent stasis-induced thrombosis. No proven occurrences of cerebral edema or hemorrhage from cortical vein occlusion have been described to date, but serious complications outside of scientific studies may be under-reported. In 1 review, the rate of major complications in patients with venous stents (2.9%) was higher than following ONSF (1.5%) but lower than in patients after CSF diversion (7.6%).[54] A complete listing of stent-related complications in IIH can be found in **Table 4**.

Fulminant Papilledema

Most patients were treated after demonstration of either failure to respond to medications or medication intolerance. However, some patients have central visual field and visual acuity loss with high-grade papilledema from the start and require a surgical intervention to stabilize or reverse vision loss at presentation, even before medications have been tried. It remains unclear whether venous sinus stenting works quickly enough to be effective in these hyperacute situations. However, venous stenting has been performed in several patients in this category. Elder and colleagues[55] placed venous stents in 4 patients with acute visual deterioration, preceded by high-volume LP (3 patients) or lumbar drain (1 patient) to temporize.[55] One patient had only mild visual acuity and field loss, and at follow-up the MD deteriorated significantly in the right eye despite resolution of papilledema. One patient descended from 4/200 OD (right eye) and 2/200 OS (left eye) to blind in both eyes, but this patient presented with optic atrophy, so there was likely little chance of recovery. The 2 other patients showed significant improvement in visual fields following stenting. Out of the 52 patients in Ahmed colleagues'[34] study, 4 presented with fulminant vision loss, but all underwent bilateral sequential ONSF prior to stenting, which could have confounded the results. In our study, 4 patients presented with Frisén grade 4 or 5 papilledema in both eyes and severe visual field loss with MD less than 10 dB in at least 1 eye.[33] All patients underwent high-volume LP before stenting. Out of 5 eyes with MD less than 10 dB, all improved by at least 4 dB, and 3 improved by greater than or equal to 9 dB. Of the 2 eyes with significant acuity loss, both improved (20/30–20/25 and 20/60–20/25^{+2}).

Table 4
Complications from venous sinus stenting

Complications	n	%
Ipsilateral headache	84	30.2
Stent thrombosis	2	0.7
Transient hearing loss	4	1.4
Restenosis	0	0.0
Allergy	2	0.7
Anaphylaxis	1	0.4
Extravasation	1	0.4
Vision loss	1	0.4
Stent migration	1	0.4
Deep vein thrombosis	1	0.4
TS thrombosis	1	0.4
SDH/ICH	4	1.4
Ataxia	0	0.0
Retroperitoneal hemorrhage	2	0.7
Femoral pseudoaneurysm	2	0.7
Urinary tract infection	1	0.4
Ruptured ovarian cyst	1	0.4
Syncope	1	0.4
Death (attributed to anesthesia)	1	0.4

Abbreviations: ICH, intracranial hemorrhage; SDH, subdural hematoma; TS, transverse sinus.

Together, these results suggest that venous stenting is a viable option even for patients with acute, severe vision loss, although greater numbers are needed to confirm this. The immediate decrease in ICP from 70 to 20 to 25 cm H_2O with stenting in a patient who was simultaneously monitored with a parenchymal ICP monitor[23] shows that, at least in some patients, stenting can produce an immediate improvement in ICP allowing stabilization or even reversal of vision loss observed in many of the published studies. **Fig. 5** shows the outcomes for a patient with fulminant visual field loss following stenting.

FUTURE DIRECTIONS

Toward a Better Stent

As venous sinus stenting for IIH becomes more readily available, it is important to highlight that the stents used for this procedure have been designed for other parts of the body with different characteristics. Most stent devices reported in the literature include stents designed for the extracranial carotid arteries, the femoral and iliac arteries, or the biliary system. As a result, these are stiff devices with high radial force necessary to oppose the wall and dilate a large artery narrowed by chronic atherosclerosis with calcifications. They also require large catheter systems for delivery. In contrast, the ideal stent for the venous sinus should be comfortable and easy to navigate through the tortuous jugular bulb and SS, delivered via a smaller catheter system, have low surface coverage to minimize the risk of compromised outflow of the cortical veins, and be long enough to cover most of the TS and SS (and thus minimize the risk of new stenosis adjacent to the stent). In addition, a

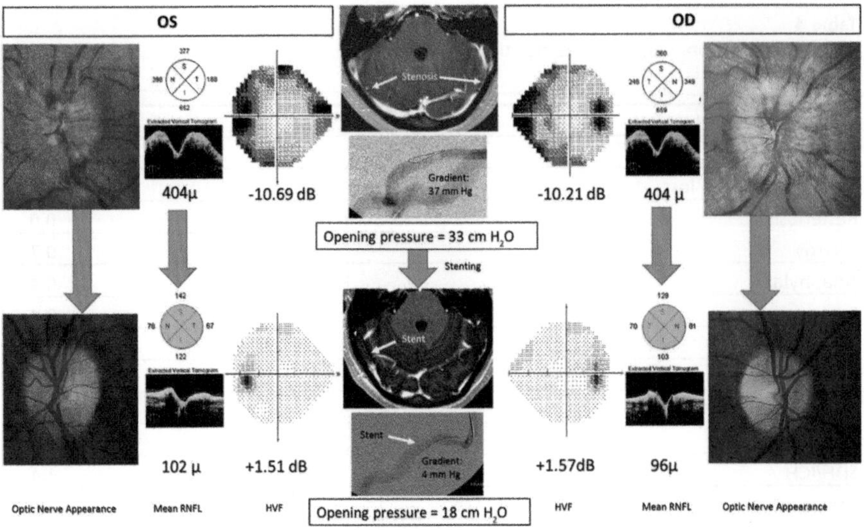

Fig. 5. A 37-year-old woman presented with headaches, pulsatile tinnitus, and TVOs. Humphrey visual fields revealed severely enlarged blind spots and arcuate defects in both eyes with MDs of −10.21 dB in the right eye and −10.69 dB in the left. Funduscopy revealed Frisén grade IV papilledema with peripapillary hemorrhages and cotton-wool spots in both eyes and OCT showed RNFL thickening to 404 μ in both eyes. MRI brain was normal but MRV showed stenosis at the TS-SS junction bilaterally. LP showed normal contents but an OP of 33 cm H_2O. There was no improvement in symptoms or papilledema within a month despite treatment with topiramate and acetazolamide. Aspirin and clopidogrel were started. Conventional venography with intravascular ultrasonography confirmed the stenosis and manometry revealed a TSG of 37 mm Hg across the right-sided stenosis. A stent was placed and the gradient reduced to 4 mm Hg. All symptoms resolved within days. At the 3-month follow-up, papilledema and visual field defects fully resolved and OCT showed normal RNFL thicknesses without atrophy. She was stable at a 1-year follow-up.

stent with less radial force would still be able to dilate the venous sinus, although it would cause less dural stretching and possibly fewer postprocedure headaches. Development of a stent with these characteristics would be a major advancement for this treatment. Video 2 shows placement of a stent at the transverse-sigmoid junction.

Intravascular Ultrasound

Intravascular ultrasonography is another important tool that can help improve the venous stent procedure by providing 360° views of the lumen of the venous sinus and therefore accurate measurement of the degree and length of the stenosis as well as information regarding the type of stenosis (intrinsic vs extrinsic). In our experience, this additional information leads to more accurate diagnosis and aids treatment planning and stent placement (**Fig. 6** and Videos 3 and 4).

LIMITATIONS

Although a review of outcomes in the patients who have received venous sinus stenting in the literature suggests both efficacy and safety, there are numerous limitations inherent in such a meta-analysis, including the varied methodology of stent

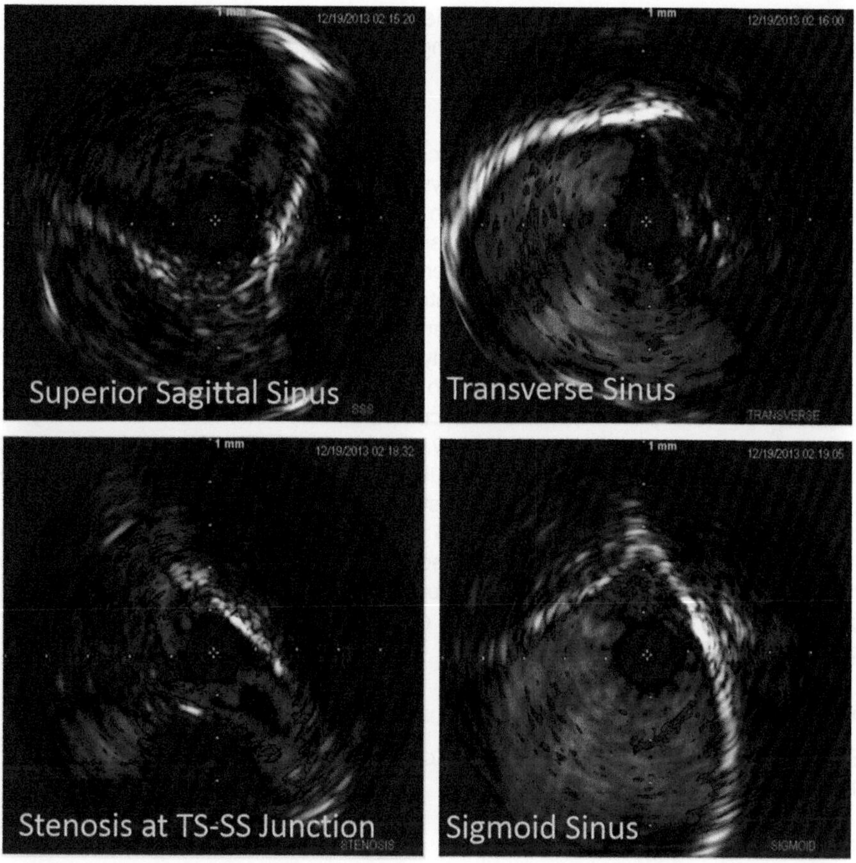

Fig. 6. Intravascular ultrasonography. Note the narrowing at the TS-SS junction (*bottom left*).

placement, follow-up times, and means of patient assessment. As mentioned, most studies were retrospective, and confounding factors likely contributed to improvement, including weight loss and concomitant medical therapy. Improvement in symptoms may have been affected by a placebo effect in some patients. Furthermore, only a few studies performed a quantitative analysis of the effect of stenting on visual fields, leaving little certainty about the success rate as measured by visual field preservation.

Although mean clinical follow-up was 21 months, the range was as short as 4 months in 1 study and on the order of weeks in some patients. Thus the long-term efficacy and complication rate of stenting remain to be fully understood. Although Ducruet and colleagues[43] aimed to remedy this with a report of 30 patients, all of whom were followed for at least 24 months, and in whom no long-term complications were reported, clinical follow-up (apart from headache outcome) was not included.

Despite these limitations, the available data are comparable, with similar data for alternative surgical therapies, albeit with much smaller patient numbers. In a review comparing 136 stented patients with 712 who underwent ONSF and 435 who underwent CSF diversion procedures, Satti and colleagues[54] found higher rates of improvement in headache, papilledema, and vision in the stenting group. These results may reflect the presence of more fulminant patients in the other 2 groups, but nevertheless argue for continued assessment of stenting as a surgical procedure for IIH.[54]

SUMMARY

The last 20 years have seen a great advancement in understanding of the contribution of venous hemodynamics to the pathophysiology of IIH. Sinus stenosis at the TS-SS junction seems to be a common finding in patients with the disease, but whether its presence is a primary cause of the disease or simply a link in a chain of events that leads to uncontrolled intracranial hypertension remains to be seen. Irrespective of the exact mechanism of its effect on ICP, stenting of VSS seems to have had a positive effect on ICP-related symptoms, papilledema, visual acuity, and ICP in those patients who underwent poststent LP, based mostly on retrospective data. The 1 uncontrolled prospective trial in the literature needs to be complimented by larger, multicenter, physician-blinded, randomized trials that compare outcomes with alternative surgical therapies and/or maximal medical therapy. As more patients undergo the procedure, complications should be reported so a full picture of its risks and benefits is elucidated. In our clinic, we present venous stenting as an experimental procedure for medically refractory IIH that seems to be effective in most cases, and discuss it in the context of alternative surgical procedures. Identifying which patients are the best candidates for venous stenting will be an important objective of future studies and it is hoped that they will lead to an even better success rate and even fewer complications.

SUPPLEMENTARY DATA

Supplementary data related to this article can be found online at http://dx.doi.org/10.1016/j.ncl.2016.08.006.

REFERENCES

1. Quincke H. Über meningitis serosa. Sammlung Klinische Vortrage (Innere Medezin 23) 1893;67:655–94.
2. Corbett JJ, Thompson HS. The rational management of idiopathic intracranial hypertension. Arch Neurol 1989;46(10):1049–51.
3. Dandy WE. Intracranial pressure without brain tumor: diagnosis and treatment. Ann Surg 1937;106(4):492–513.
4. Chen L, Elias G, Yostos MP, et al. Pathways of cerebrospinal fluid outflow: a deeper understanding of resorption. Neuroradiology 2015;57(2):139–47.
5. Dinkin M, Moss HE. Should magnetic resonance venography be performed routinely in all patients undergoing evaluation for idiopathic intracranial hypertension? J Neuroophthalmol 2015;35(4):431–7.
6. Farb RI, Vanek I, Scott JN, et al. Idiopathic intracranial hypertension: the prevalence and morphology of sinovenous stenosis. Neurology 2003;60(9):1418–24.
7. King JO, Mitchell PJ, Thomson KR, et al. Cerebral venography and manometry in idiopathic intracranial hypertension. Neurology 1995;45(12):2224–8.
8. NORDIC Idiopathic Intracranial Hypertension Study Group Writing Committee, Wall M, McDermott MP, Kieburtz KD, et al. Effect of acetazolamide on visual function in patients with idiopathic intracranial hypertension and mild visual loss: the Idiopathic Intracranial Hypertension Treatment Trial. JAMA 2014;311(16):1641–51.

9. Wall M, George D. Idiopathic intracranial hypertension. A prospective study of 50 patients. Brain 1991;114(Pt 1A):155–80.
10. Thambisetty M, Lavin PJ, Newman NJ, et al. Fulminant idiopathic intracranial hypertension. Neurology 2007;68(3):229–32.
11. Banta JT, Farris BK. Pseudotumor cerebri and optic nerve sheath decompression. Ophthalmology 2000;107(10):1907–12.
12. Menger RP, Connor DE, Thakur JD, et al. A comparison of lumboperitoneal and ventriculoperitoneal shunting for idiopathic intracranial hypertension: an analysis of economic impact and complications using the Nationwide Inpatient Sample. Neurosurg Focus 2014;37(5):E4.
13. Higgins JNP, Owler BK, Cousins C, et al. Venous sinus stenting for refractory benign intracranial hypertension. Lancet 2002;359(9302):228–30.
14. Higgins JNP, Cousins C, Owler BK, et al. Idiopathic intracranial hypertension: 12 cases treated by venous sinus stenting. J Neurol Neurosurg Psychiatry 2003; 74(12):1662–6.
15. Ogungbo B, Roy D, Gholkar A, et al. Endovascular stenting of the transverse sinus in a patient presenting with benign intracranial hypertension. Br J Neurosurg 2003;17(6):565–8.
16. Rajpal S, Niemann DB, Turk AS. Transverse venous sinus stent placement as treatment for benign intracranial hypertension in a young male: case report and review of the literature. J Neurosurg 2005;102(3 Suppl):342–6.
17. Paquet C, Poupardin M, Boissonnot M, et al. Efficacy of unilateral stenting in idiopathic intracranial hypertension with bilateral venous sinus stenosis: a case report. Eur Neurol 2008;60(1):47–8.
18. Crosa R, Marabotto O, Meehroff G, et al. Pseudotumor cerebri: a new door opens for treatment. Interv Neuroradiol 2007;13(2):145–51.
19. Arac A, Lee M, Steinberg GK, et al. Efficacy of endovascular stenting in dural venous sinus stenosis for the treatment of idiopathic intracranial hypertension. Neurosurg Focus 2009;27(5):E14.
20. Zheng H, Zhou M, Zhao B, et al. Pseudotumor cerebri syndrome and giant arachnoid granulation: treatment with venous sinus stenting. J Vasc Interv Radiol 2010; 21(6):927–9.
21. Crawford A, McGrath NM. Hearing loss after lumbar puncture. J Clin Neurosci 2010;17(1):149–52.
22. Spilberg G, Wajnberg E, Casparetto E, et al. Endovascular treatment of idiopathic intracranial hypertension. Pakistani Journal of Radiology 2010;20(1):23–6.
23. Fargen KM, Velat GJ, Lewis SB, et al. Concomitant intracranial pressure monitoring during venous sinus stenting for intracranial hypertension secondary to venous sinus stenosis. J Neurointerv Surg 2013;5(4):e22.
24. Ding D, Starke RM, Durst CR, et al. Venous stenting with concurrent intracranial pressure monitoring for the treatment of pseudotumor cerebri. Neurosurg Focus 2014;37(1 Suppl):1.
25. Donnet A, Metellus P, Levrier O, et al. Endovascular treatment of idiopathic intracranial hypertension: clinical and radiologic outcome of 10 consecutive patients. Neurology 2008;70(8):641–7.
26. Bussière M, Falero R, Nicolle D, et al. Unilateral transverse sinus stenting of patients with idiopathic intracranial hypertension. AJNR Am J Neuroradiol 2010; 31(4):645–50.
27. Albuquerque FC, Dashti SR, Hu YC, et al. Intracranial venous sinus stenting for benign intracranial hypertension: clinical indications, technique, and preliminary results. World Neurosurg 2011;75(5–6):648–52 [discussion 592–5].

28. Kumpe DA, Bennett JL, Seinfeld J, et al. Dural sinus stent placement for idiopathic intracranial hypertension. J Neurosurg 2012;116(3):538–48.
29. Fields JD, Javedani PP, Falardeau J, et al. Dural venous sinus angioplasty and stenting for the treatment of idiopathic intracranial hypertension. J Neurointerv Surg 2013;5(1):62–8.
30. Radvany MG, Solomon D, Nijjar S, et al. Visual and neurological outcomes following endovascular stenting for pseudotumor cerebri associated with transverse sinus stenosis. J Neuroophthalmol 2013;33(2):117–22.
31. Teleb MS, Cziep ME, Issa M, et al. Stenting and angioplasty for idiopathic intracranial hypertension: a case series with clinical, angiographic, ophthalmological, complication, and pressure reporting. J Neuroimaging 2015;25(1):72–80.
32. Smith KA, Peterson JC, Arnold PM, et al. A case series of dural venous sinus stenting in idiopathic intracranial hypertension: association of outcomes with optical coherence tomography. Int J Neurosci 2016;1–9.
33. Dinkin M, Patsalides A. Venous sinus stenting in idiopathic intracranial hypertension: results of a prospective trial. J Neuroophthalmol 2016;0:1–9.
34. Ahmed RM, Wilkinson M, Parker GD, et al. Transverse sinus stenting for idiopathic intracranial hypertension: a review of 52 patients and of model predictions. AJNR Am J Neuroradiol 2011;32(8):1408–14.
35. King JO, Mitchell PJ, Thomson KR, et al. Manometry combined with cervical puncture in idiopathic intracranial hypertension. Neurology 2002;58(1):26–30.
36. Rohr A, Dörner L, Stingele R, et al. Reversibility of venous sinus obstruction in idiopathic intracranial hypertension. AJNR Am J Neuroradiol 2007;28(4):656–9.
37. Bono F, Giliberto C, Mastrandrea C, et al. Transverse sinus stenoses persist after normalization of the CSF pressure in IIH. Neurology 2005;65(7):1090–3.
38. Connor SEJ, Siddiqui MA, Stewart VR, et al. The relationship of transverse sinus stenosis to bony groove dimensions provides an insight into the aetiology of idiopathic intracranial hypertension. Neuroradiology 2008;50(12):999–1004.
39. Kelly LP, Saindane AM, Bruce BB, et al. Does bilateral transverse cerebral venous sinus stenosis exist in patients without increased intracranial pressure? Clin Neurol Neurosurg 2013;115(8):1215–9.
40. Stevens SA, Stimpson J, Lakin WD, et al. A model for idiopathic intracranial hypertension and associated pathological ICP wave-forms. IEEE Trans Biomed Eng 2008;55(2 Pt 1):388–98.
41. He C, Ji X, Wang L, et al. Endovascular treatment for venous sinus stenosis in idiopathic intracranial hypertension. Zhonghua Yi Xue Za Zhi 2012;92(11): 748–51 [in Chinese].
42. Lazzaro MA, Darkhabani Z, Remler BF, et al. Venous sinus pulsatility and the potential role of dural incompetence in idiopathic intracranial hypertension. Neurosurgery 2012;71(4):877–83.
43. Ducruet AF, Crowley RW, McDougall CG, et al. Long-term patency of venous sinus stents for idiopathic intracranial hypertension. J Neurointerv Surg 2014;6(3): 238–42.
44. Riggeal BD, Bruce BB, Saindane AM, et al. Clinical course of idiopathic intracranial hypertension with transverse sinus stenosis. Neurology 2013;80(3):289–95.
45. Saindane AM, Bruce BB, Riggeal BD, et al. Association of MRI findings and visual outcome in idiopathic intracranial hypertension. AJR Am J Roentgenol 2013; 201(2):412–8.
46. Ahmed RM, Parker GD, Halmagyi GM. Letters to the editor: stenting and idiopathic intracranial hypertension. J Neurosurg 2012;117(6):1205 [author reply: 1205–6].

47. Lai LT, Danesh-Meyer HV, Kaye AH. Visual outcomes and headache following interventions for idiopathic intracranial hypertension. J Clin Neurosci 2014;21(10):1670–8.
48. Karam EZ, Hedges TR. Optical coherence tomography of the retinal nerve fibre layer in mild papilloedema and pseudopapilloedema. Br J Ophthalmol 2005;89(3):294–8.
49. Alessi G, Levrier O, Conrath J, et al. Optical coherence tomography in following up papilledema in idiopathic intracranial hypertension treated with lateral sinus stent placement. J Fr Ophtalmol 2010;33(9):637–48 [in French].
50. Fonseca AC, Albuquerque L, Ferro JM. Reversible bilateral sensorineural hearing loss in a woman with cerebral venous thrombosis. J Neurol 2008;255(11):1825–6.
51. Ahmed R, Friedman DI, Halmagyi GM. Stenting of the transverse sinuses in idiopathic intracranial hypertension. J Neuroophthalmol 2011;31(4):374–80.
52. Li G, Warner M, Lang BH, et al. Epidemiology of anesthesia-related mortality in the United States, 1999-2005. Anesthesiology 2009;110(4):759–65.
53. Levitt MR, Albuquerque FC, Ducruet AF, et al. Venous sinus stenting for idiopathic intracranial hypertension is not associated with cortical venous occlusion. J Neurointerv Surg 2016. http://dx.doi.org/10.1136/neurintsurg-2015-011692.
54. Satti SR, Leishangthem L, Chaudry MI. Meta-analysis of CSF diversion procedures and dural venous sinus stenting in the setting of medically refractory idiopathic intracranial hypertension. AJNR Am J Neuroradiol 2015;36(10):1899–904.
55. Elder BD, Rory Goodwin C, Kosztowski TA, et al. Venous sinus stenting is a valuable treatment for fulminant idiopathic intracranial hypertension. J Clin Neurosci 2015;22(4):685–9.

Update on the Management of Central Retinal Artery Occlusion

Michael Dattilo, MD, PhD[a,b], Valérie Biousse, MD[a,b,c,*], Nancy J. Newman, MD[a,b,c,d]

KEYWORDS

- Central retinal artery occlusion • Branch retinal artery occlusion • Stroke • Ischemia • Management • Treatment • Thrombolysis

KEY POINTS

- Acute central retinal artery occlusion (CRAO) and branch retinal artery occlusion (BRAO) are the ocular equivalent of a cerebral infarction in the anterior circulation.
- The risk factors for a CRAO or a BRAO and acute cerebral ischemia are very similar.
- Patients with acute CRAO and BRAO need to be evaluated emergently in a stroke center similar to patients with cerebral ischemia.
- Up to 24% of patients with acute retinal ischemia have concomitant cerebral infarctions on brain diffusion-weighted MRI.
- Because no current therapeutic intervention has been shown to improve visual outcome compared with the natural history of CRAO, management of CRAO should be focused on secondary prevention of vascular events, such as cerebral ischemia, myocardial infarction, and cardiovascular death.

Disclosure Statement: M. Dattilo has no disclosures. V. Biousse and N. Newman are consultants for GenSight Biologics. N. Newman is a consultant for Santhera Pharmaceuticals. V. Biousse and N. Newman are supported in part by an unrestricted departmental grant (Department of Ophthalmology) from Research to Prevent Blindness, Inc, New York, by NIH/NEI core grant P30-EY06360 (Department of Ophthalmology, Emory University School of Medicine), and by NIH/NINDS (RO1NSO89694).

[a] Department of Ophthalmology, Emory University School of Medicine, 1365-B Clifton Road, Northeast, Atlanta, GA 30322, USA; [b] Neuro-Ophthalmology, Emory Eye Center, 1365-B Clifton Road, Northeast, Atlanta, GA 30322, USA; [c] Department of Neurology, Emory University School of Medicine, 12 Executive Park Drive, Northeast, Atlanta, GA 30329, USA; [d] Department of Neurological Surgery, Emory University School of Medicine, Atlanta, GA 30322, USA

* Corresponding author. Neuro-Ophthalmology, Emory Eye Center, 1365-B Clifton Road, Northeast, Atlanta, GA 30322.

E-mail address: vbiouss@emory.edu

Neurol Clin 35 (2017) 83–100
http://dx.doi.org/10.1016/j.ncl.2016.08.013

neurologic.theclinics.com

BACKGROUND

Central retinal artery occlusion (CRAO) was first described in 1859 in a patient with endocarditis[1] and is caused by partial or complete obstruction of the central retinal artery (CRA) leading to retinal ischemia (**Figs. 1** and **2**). The CRA originates from the ophthalmic artery, which is the first branch of the internal carotid artery. The CRA and its branches supply blood to the inner retina, including the macula and fovea. Occlusion of a branch of the CRA causes a branch retinal artery occlusion (BRAO) (**Fig. 3**). In approximately 15% to 30% of the population, a cilioretinal artery is present, originating from the posterior ciliary circulation and not the CRA, often supplying part of the macula and fovea (**Fig. 4**).[2–4] Because the cilioretinal artery does not originate from the CRA, it is spared in a CRAO. If the cilioretinal artery supplies the fovea, central visual acuity may be near normal (20/50 or better) following a CRAO, whereas peripheral vision in the effected eye will be severely impaired (see **Fig. 4**).[3,5]

CRAO and BRAO are most often embolic, and the causes and risk factors are similar to those of patients with cerebrovascular ischemic events; these are classically referred

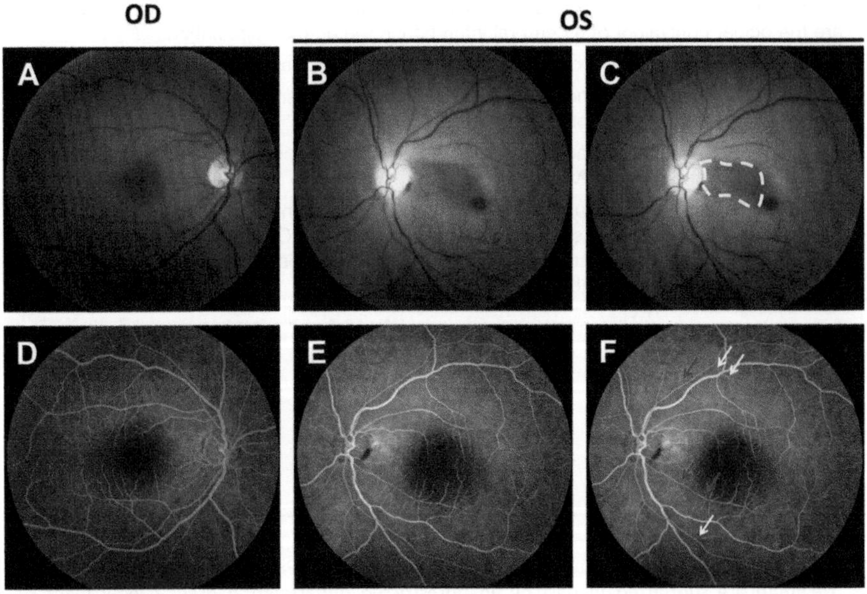

Fig. 1. Left CRAO with cilioretinal artery sparing. Color fundus photographs (*A–C*) and retinal fluorescein angiography (*D–F*) in acute CRAO. (*A*) Color fundus photograph of the right eye (OD) showing a normal appearing fundus. (*B*) Color fundus photographs of the left eye (OS) showing a CRAO with cilioretinal artery sparing. Compared with the right eye, the fundus of the left eye has a white hue, indicating inner retinal edema. The papillomacular bundle is perfused by patent cilioretinal arteries. (*C*) Same photograph as in (*B*) outlining the area perfused by the cilioretinal arteries (*area within the yellow lines*). Retinal edema is seen outside of the area perfused by the cilioretinal arteries. (*D*) Fluorescein angiography of the normal right eye taken 59 seconds from the injection of fluorescein dye into the patient's arm. The retinal arteries are of normal caliber and the retina is well perfused. (*E*) Fluorescein angiogram of the left eye taken 46 seconds after injection of fluorescein dye. The retinal arteries in the left eye are attenuated as compared with the retinal arteries in the right eye (*red arrows in* [*F*]), and areas of discontinuity in the retinal arteries of the left eye are also noted (*yellow arrows in* [*F*]).

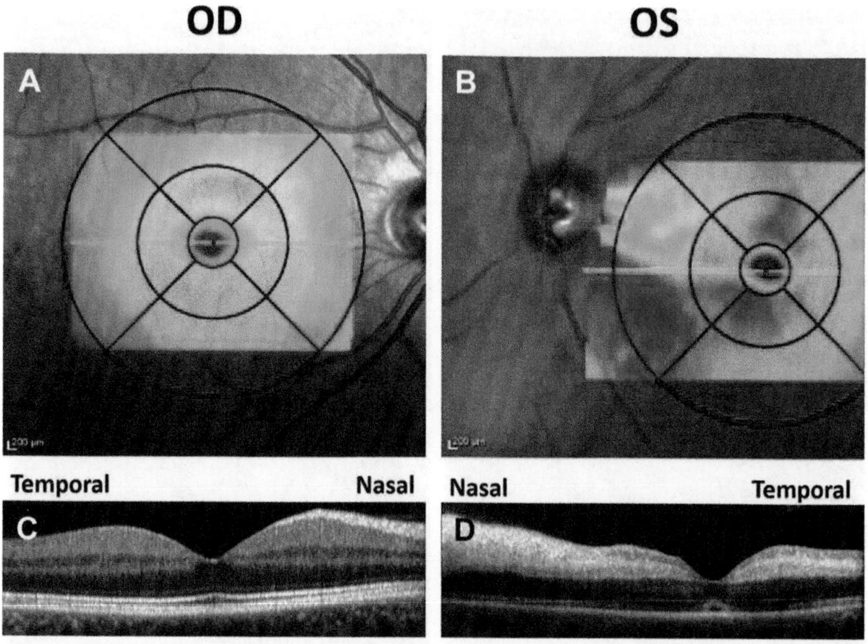

Fig. 2. Optical coherence tomography (OCT) of the macula in acute CRAO (from the patient in **Fig. 1**). (*A, B*) En face OCT images of the macula of the right eye (*A*) and left eye (*B*) with superimposed pseudocolored thickness maps. (*A*) OCT of the right macula showing normal macular thickness. (*B*) OCT of the left macula showing macular thickening (*red areas*) consistent with retinal edema seen in **Fig. 1**B, C. The area of the papillomacular bundle is green (normal thickness) corresponding to the area perfused by the cilioretinal arteries (see **Fig. 1**B, C). (*C, D*) OCT line scan of the right eye (*C*) and left eye (*D*) corresponding to the horizontal green line in (*A*) and (*B*), respectively. (*C*) Normal retinal thickness and architecture in the right eye. (*D*) Increased nasal retinal thickness (edema) is seen.

to as nonarteritic CRAO and BRAO. Rarely, CRAO and BRAO can result from vasculitis, particularly in patients with giant cell arteritis (GCA) (arteritic CRAO).[3,6–9] Nonarteritic transient CRAO is the ocular equivalent of a cerebral transient ischemic attack (TIA). Although it is not specifically discussed in this review, acute management of transient retinal ischemia should be similar to that of patients with permanent retinal ischemia.[10]

For the remainder of this review, the terms *CRAO* and *BRAO* are used to refer to nonarteritic CRAO or BRAO, respectively.

INCIDENCE OF CENTRAL RETINAL ARTERY OCCLUSION

The incidence of all nonarteritic forms of CRAO is approximately 1 to 2 in 100,000, and CRAO accounts for approximately 1 in 10,000 outpatient ophthalmology visits.[11–13] The incidence of CRAO increases with age and may be as high as 10 in 100,000 in patients older than 80 years, likely because of the higher prevalence of cardiovascular disease in this age group.[12,14]

DIAGNOSIS OF CENTRAL RETINAL ARTERY OCCLUSION

CRAO typically presents as sudden, painless loss of vision and/or visual field in the involved eye. Visual acuity following a CRAO varies greatly, ranging from near normal

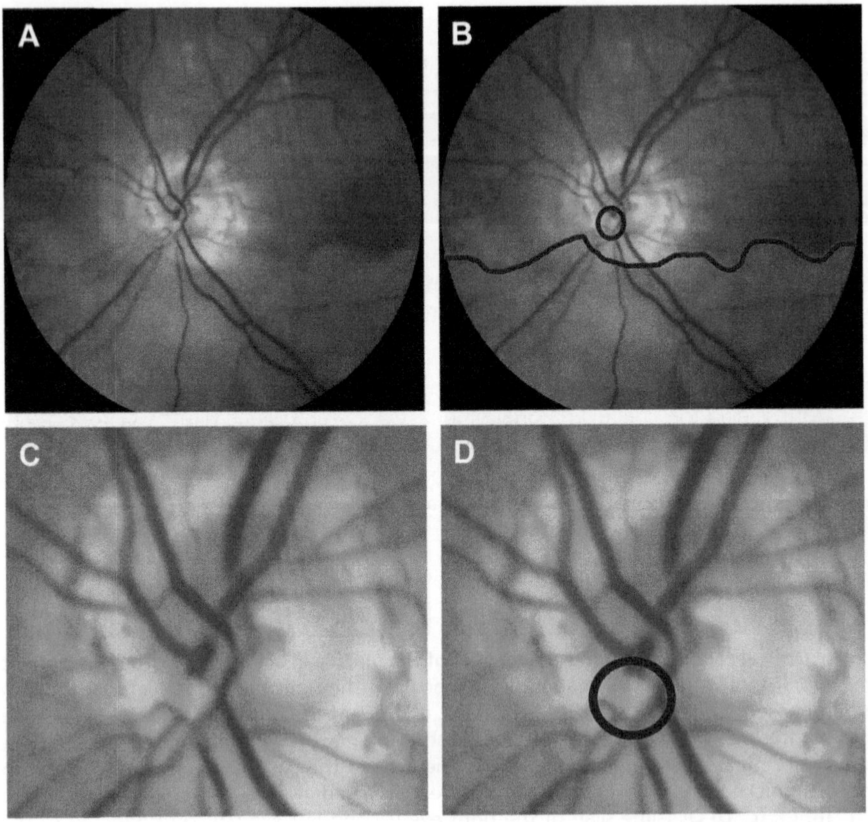

Fig. 3. Left inferior BRAO. Color fundus photographs of the left retina (*A, B*) and a magnified view of the left optic nerve (*C, D*). (*A*) Color fundus photograph of the left eye showing an occlusion in an inferior branch of the central retinal artery and associated inferior retinal whitening suggesting retinal edema. (*B*) Same photograph as in (*A*). The blue circle denotes the location of the occlusion in the inferior branch of the CRA. Retinal whitening (edema) is seen below the blue line. (*C*) Magnified view of the left optic nerve showing an occlusion in an inferior branch of the CRA overlying the optic disc. (*D*) Same photograph as in (*C*). The blue circle shows the occlusion in the branch retinal artery.

visual acuity in the presence of a cilioretinal artery sparing the fovea to counting fingers or worse vision in most patients. Indeed, in a study of 260 eyes with a CRAO, 74% had a presenting visual acuity of counting fingers or worse and most patients with better visual acuity had a cilioretinal artery that perfused or partially perfused the fovea.[7] Color vision is decreased in parallel to the decrease in visual acuity, and there is a relative afferent pupillary defect. The classic retinal findings seen on funduscopic examination include retinal edema (evident as retinal whitening), a cherry red spot (seen as a pink or red fovea due to the presence of normal underlying choroidal circulation in the fovea where there is only a very thin nerve fiber layer), retinal arteriolar attenuation, slow segmental blood flow in retinal arterioles (known as box-carring), and a normal optic nerve.[2,15] Emboli in the CRA or its branches may be visible. There is no optic disc edema unless the ophthalmic artery is occluded, in which case there is typically no visible cherry red spot. Visible retinal findings may not be present or obvious in the acute setting and may take several hours to develop (see **Fig. 1**).[2,9,15] Imaging

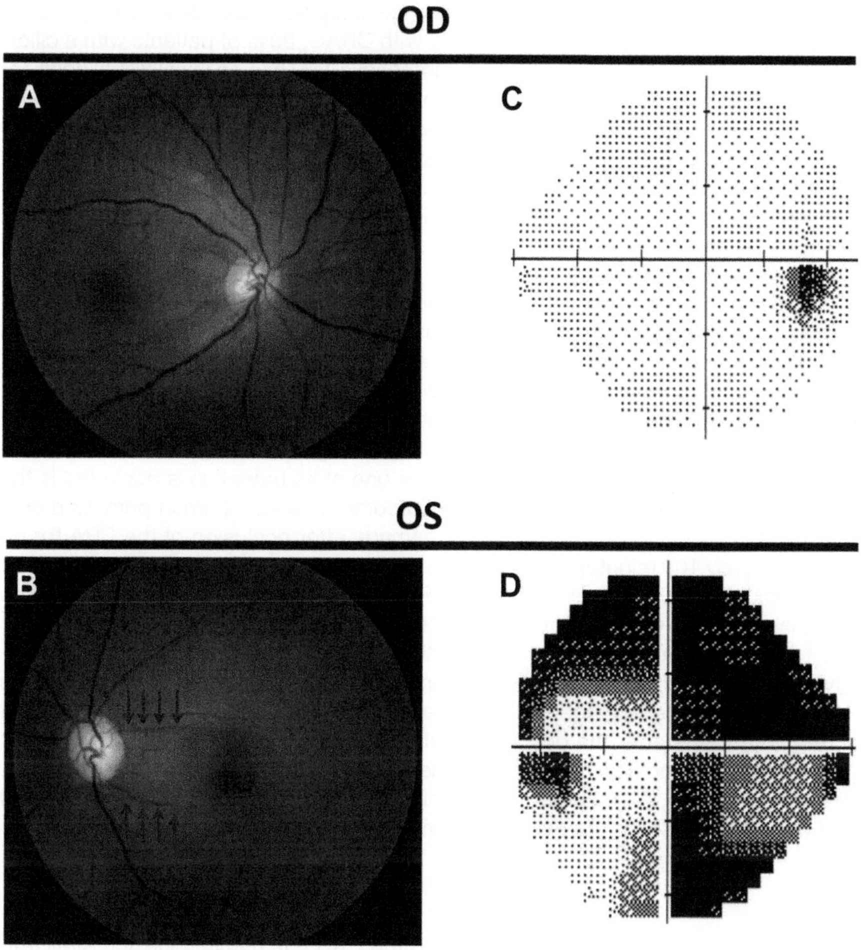

Fig. 4. Left CRAO with cilioretinal artery sparing. (*A*) Color fundus photograph of the normal right eye. (*B*) Color fundus photograph of the left eye showing a CRAO with perfused cilioretinal arteries (*blue arrows*). The remainder of the retinal arterioles is severely attenuated. Visual acuity in the left eye was 20/40. (*C*) Normal Humphrey visual field from the right eye. (*D*) Left eye Humphrey visual field showing marked visual field deficits despite near normal visual acuity, due to patent cilioretinal arteries, in the left eye.

modalities, such as optical coherence tomography (OCT) or retinal fluorescein angiography, may facilitate the diagnosis of a retinal artery occlusion (CRAO or BRAO) in unclear cases or when the expected examination findings are very subtle or absent. OCT can detect retinal edema acutely and disruption or thinning of inner retinal layers once the edema has resolved (see **Fig. 2**).[16] Retinal fluorescein angiography may demonstrate delayed or absent retinal arteriolar blood flow (see **Fig. 1**E).[9,17]

VISUAL OUTCOME

CRAO is classically associated with severe visual loss. The visual outcome in CRAO, although typically poor, is variable and depends on several factors, including the length of time the CRA is occluded, the presence of a patent cilioretinal artery, and the type of embolus.[5] In a study of 244 patients with CRAO, 20% of patients with a cilioretinal artery and only 1 patient without a cilioretinal artery had an initial visual acuity of 20/40 or better. However, 60.0% with a cilioretinal artery (not reaching the fovea) and 93.2% without a cilioretinal artery had an initial visual acuity of counting fingers or worse. In those patients who had an initial visual acuity of counting fingers or worse, 47% with a cilioretinal artery and 16% without a cilioretinal artery showed some improvement in visual acuity, whereas the final visual acuity was worse than the presenting visual acuity in 6% with a cilioretinal artery and 8% without a cilioretinal artery.[5,7] With respect to visual field defects, approximately 20% to 25% of patients with a central scotoma on presentation had improvement in their central scotoma, irrespective of the presence of a cilioretinal artery.[7] These data suggest that most patients with a CRAO do not demonstrate spontaneous improvement in visual function and continue to have profound visual dysfunction in the involved eye; however, the presence of a cilioretinal artery is associated with a higher likelihood of initial good vision and subsequent improvement in visual acuity (see **Fig. 4**).

It is likely that the length of time the CRA or one of its branches is occluded is the most important determinant of final visual outcome. In a non–human primate model of CRAO, there was no detectable retinal damage after occlusion of the CRA for up to approximately 100 minutes; however, massive, irreversible retinal damage occurred after approximately 240 minutes of occlusion. Between 100 minutes and 240 minutes of occlusion of the CRA, variable amounts of permanent retinal dysfunction were seen.[18,19] These studies strongly suggest that the duration of retinal ischemia positively correlates with the likelihood of improvement in visual function following a CRAO. Similar to the management of an acute cerebral infarction, there is likely a discrete time frame after the occurrence of a CRAO when therapeutic interventions to restore retinal blood flow may have a beneficial effect on visual outcome. Therefore, at least theoretically, the sooner a diagnosis is made, therapy instituted, and retinal blood flow reestablished, the better the chance for visual recovery.[5,18,19]

CAUSE

Any process that obstructs the blood flow to the CRA can cause a CRAO. Similar to cerebral infarctions in the anterior circulation, the most common cause of CRAO and BRAO is an embolus in the affected artery. Such emboli originate most often from the ipsilateral internal carotid artery, followed by the aortic arch, and the heart. Thrombosis of the CRAO from a hypercoagulable state or vasculitis (such as in giant cell arteritis) is less common but must be considered when the initial workup fails to identify a source of emboli.[6,8,9,20,21] When retinal emboli are seen on funduscopic examination, the evaluation must focus on looking for a source of emboli. Not surprisingly, there is a strong correlation between CRAO and the presence of cardiovascular risk factors, such as hypertension, atherosclerosis, and diabetes, similar to patients with cerebral infarctions.[2,8,14,22–24] In the patient population included in the European Assessment Group for Lysis in the Eye (EAGLE) trial, 73% of 77 patients with CRAO had arterial hypertension, 40% had at least a 70% stenosis of a carotid artery (with most having ipsilateral carotid artery stenosis), 22% had coronary artery disease, 20% had atrial fibrillation, and 17% had valvular heart disease. Although most of these patients had known cardiovascular risk factors, at least 1 new cardiovascular risk factor was identified at the time of the CRAO in 78% of patients, with hypercholesterolemia and carotid artery stenosis being the most frequent newly diagnosed cardiovascular risk factors.[22] Although there is a strong association between CRAO and carotid atheroma, in the appropriate clinical context and patient demographic, other causes of CRAO aside from atheromatous disease must also be considered, including carotid dissections and cardiac sources of emboli.

The presence of facial pain or headache associated with a CRAO should raise concern for an ipsilateral carotid artery dissection, either spontaneous or following neck trauma or chiropractic neck manipulation.[25,26] These patients often have a Horner syndrome ipsilateral to the CRAO.[25] Initial diagnostic studies should be focused on evaluating both the extracranial and intracranial carotid arteries, ideally with a computed tomography angiogram or magnetic resonance angiography (MRA) (**Fig. 5**). In addition, GCA should be considered in any patient older than 50 years who presents with a CRAO, especially if there is associated jaw pain, temporal headaches, or tenderness on palpation around the temporal artery.

In addition to systemic risk factors, certain ocular conditions, such as acutely elevated intraocular pressure (IOP), as is seen in some forms of glaucoma, and the presence of preretinal arterial loops and optic nerve head drusen are associated with the development of CRAO. These conditions presumably cause a CRAO by decreasing ocular perfusion across the optic nerve head.[27,28] Perioperative CRAO may be precipitated by sustained ocular compression in some patients undergoing spine surgery in the prone position.[29,30] Rarely, acute CRAO can occur after dental or facial cosmetic procedures when drugs or filling materials are inadvertently injected in a facial vessel.[31]

MORBIDITY AND MORTALITY

CRAO is associated with a high degree of morbidity and mortality due to both the direct complications (permanent, severe vision loss) and the immediate and long-term ocular and systemic risks associated with CRAO.[23,32–36]

CRAO causes severe unilateral vision loss, either because of decreased visual acuity, a markedly reduced visual field, or both, which leads to decreased independence

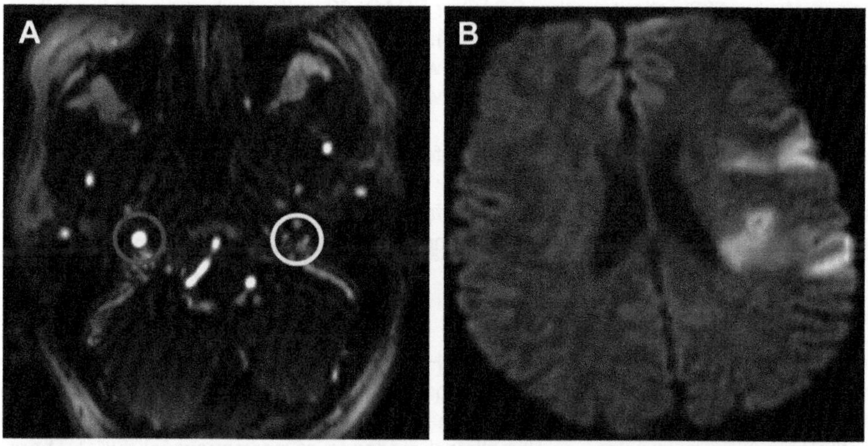

Fig. 5. Cerebral ischemia in acute CRAO (brain MRI from the patient in **Fig. 1**). (*A*) MRA of the neck showing normal filling of the right internal carotid artery (*red circle*) and absent filling of the left intracranial internal carotid (*yellow circle*) due to a left internal carotid artery dissection. (*B*) Brain diffusion-weighted imaging MRI showing a cerebral infarction in the left middle cerebral artery territory secondary to the left internal carotid artery dissection.

and quality of life and possibly institutional care.[36] Additionally, these patients need to be monitored closely by an ophthalmologist for the development of ocular neovascularization, which can occur as early as 2 weeks following a CRAO and lead to further severe vision loss.[37] Anterior segment neovascularization from chronic ocular ischemia can lead to neovascular glaucoma and markedly elevated IOP, ocular pain, and rapidly deteriorating visual acuity. Posterior segment (retinal) neovascularization can lead to vitreous hemorrhage and retinal detachment. If ocular neovascularization is detected, referral to a vitreoretinal specialist is necessary for treatment to attempt to prevent further vision loss. The visual dysfunction from a CRAO also places patients at a higher risk for falls and subsequent hip fractures, further decreasing independence and quality of life.

In addition to the immediate decrease in quality of life due to severe visual impairment from a CRAO, the development of a CRAO is associated with a higher incidence of having had a recent prior ischemic event (myocardial infarction [MI] or cerebral infarction) and a higher risk of a subsequent MI or cerebral infarction; the highest risk of a subsequent cerebral infarction occurs within the first week following a CRAO.[8,22–24,28,34,35,38,39] Indeed, among the 77 patients with CRAO included in the EAGLE study, 15 patients (19.5%) experienced either a stroke or a TIA. Five had strokes within 1 month of the CRAO, and 4 of those 5 were found to have significant carotid artery stenosis ipsilateral to the CRAO.[22] In addition, a population-based study in Taiwan reported a 2.7 times higher rate of stroke within the first 3 years in patients with a CRAO compared with matched controls, with the highest incidence of stroke occurring within the first month after the CRAO.[40] It has been reported that the stroke rate following a CRAO is as high as 13% in the first year and as much as 10 times higher than in the general population during the first 3.5 years following a CRAO. The increased risk of stroke may persist for up to 10 years following the CRAO.[35,40] In addition to an increased risk of stroke following a CRAO, cardiovascular mortality (MI or vascular death) is also high following a CRAO; some studies suggest that cardiovascular ischemic events may occur more frequently and represent a higher source of mortality in patients following a CRAO than stroke.[22,32,34] Indeed, in a prospective cohort study of 98 patients with a CRAO or BRAO, 29 patients died during the follow-up period (average follow-up of 4.2 years).[32] One person died of cerebral ischemia, and more than half of the deaths (59%) were due to a coronary event; the 5-year risk of death from a coronary event following a CRAO was 24.0% compared with 11.7% for cerebral ischemia.[32]

Therefore, CRAO may be the initial manifestation of an underlying systemic disease that places patients at a significantly higher risk than the general population for a subsequent ischemic event (MI or cerebral infarction), further decreasing independence and quality of life and increasing patient mortality.

MANAGEMENT

In 2013, the American Heart Association (AHA) and American Stroke Association (ASA) published a consensus statement defining central nervous system infarction (stroke) as "brain, spinal cord, or retinal cell death attributable to ischemia, based on neuropathological, neuroimaging, and/or clinical evidence of permanent injury."[41] Therefore, a CRAO is a stroke equivalent and is both an ophthalmologic and medical emergency. It should prompt systematic immediate referral to the nearest certified stroke center to prevent or minimize the risk of further ischemic complications, such as an MI or cerebral infarction.[6,7,10,34,35,39] Unfortunately, in a survey performed in 2009 in the state of Georgia, only approximately 35% of ophthalmologists indicated that they refer patients to emergency departments for further workup and risk stratification after diagnosing an acute CRAO.[42]

The ideal patient disposition obviously varies based on local resources, but immediate evaluation in an emergency care center affiliated with a certified stroke center allows for effective, rapid workup and consultation with a stroke neurologist. Depending on the results of the workup, which is typically performed within 24 hours, patients may be discharged with secondary prevention measures and a follow-up with a stroke neurologist or may be admitted to a stroke unit for immediate treatment of a major cause, such as carotid atheromatous stenosis, carotid dissection, or a cardiac source of embolization (see **Fig. 5**). Indeed, as emphasized by the AHA and the ASA, as well as numerous international stroke agencies, patients with an acute CRAO or BRAO must be evaluated similarly to patients with acute cerebral ischemia. The same recommendations apply to patients with transient retinal ischemia.[41]

All patients, if not contraindicated, should have an immediate MRI of the brain with diffusion-weighted imaging (DWI) to look for concurrent cerebral ischemia, even patients without any neurologic symptoms. In 3 retrospective studies, it was reported that between 23% and 24% of patients with acute retinal ischemia (CRAO, BRAO, or transient monocular visual loss) have concurrent acute small cerebral infarctions as determined by brain MRI (**Table 1**).[2,10,21,33,43–45] Most patients in these studies did not have any other focal neurologic deficits to suggest acute cerebral ischemia at the time of presentation. It is well established that such silent infarctions bear a high risk of future stroke. In the subgroup of patients with acute retinal ischemia and acute silent cerebral infarctions, a major cause for strokes is frequently identified, most often causes requiring urgent treatment to prevent subsequent strokes.[33,44,45]

The stroke workup performed in patients with CRAO must focus on assessing for the presence of an underlying source of emboli, as occlusion of the CRA by an embolus is the most common cause of CRAO. In addition to immediate brain imaging with DWI, vascular imaging of the carotid arteries and aortic arch is performed urgently, usually by MRA of the neck and head at the time of the brain MRI. A thorough evaluation for cardiovascular risk factors, including electrocardiogram and echocardiogram (ideally transesophageal), blood pressure, and cardiac monitoring (which can replace Holter monitoring when patients' workup is performed over 24 hours in a stroke center) should systematically be performed in all patients with a CRAO.[22] In younger patients with no identified cause, further evaluation could be performed, including tests for hypercoagulable conditions, such as factor V Leiden deficiency or prothrombin (20,210) gene mutations, protein C and S deficiency, antithrombin III deficiency, hyperhomocysteinemia, the presence of antiphospholipid antibodies; factor VIII excess, hyperviscosity; vasculo-occlusive disorders, such as sickle cell disease; and rheumatologic systemic inflammatory disorders; and search for the use of certain medications, such as nasal vasoconstrictive agents and the use of illicit substances, such as intravenous (IV) drugs and cocaine.[27,46]

GCA must also be considered in any patient older than 50 years who presents with an acute CRAO.[2] Patients should be asked about systemic symptoms associated with giant cell arteritis, such as headaches and jaw claudication; inflammatory markers, such as erythrocyte sedimentation rate and C-reactive protein, should be obtained. A high clinical suspicion for GCA should prompt a temporal artery biopsy, irrespective of the laboratory results.[2,3] If GCA is confirmed, patients need to be treated with high-dose IV steroids followed by a slow oral prednisone taper (beginning at 1 mg/kg) to prevent further vision loss and systemic complications.[47,48]

Table 1
Summary of 3 studies evaluating brain imaging in patients with acute retinal ischemia

Study	Patients	Clinical Presentation	Workup	MRI Results	Correlation with Abnormal DWI MRI
Helenius et al,[33] 2012 (Boston)	2000–2008 129 Consecutive Aged 64 ±16 y Retrospective Systematic evaluation	Isolated TMVL: 66 Isolated BRAO/CRAO: 46 Neuro sx + TMVL: 8 Neuro sx + BRAO/CRAO: 9	≤7 d of VL Standard stroke workup	DWI+ in 31 of 129 (24%) Same vascular territory as visual loss in 28 of 31 Small, multiple infarctions	Neuro sx+ Permanent VL > TMVL Identified cause Embolic cause
Lee et al,[45] 2014 (Korea)	2005–2012 33 Consecutive Aged 58 ±14 y Retrospective Systematic evaluation	BRAO: 15 CRAO: 18 + Neuro sx: 5	≤7 d of VL Standard stroke workup	DWI+ in 8 of 33 (24.2%) Same vascular territory as visual loss in 8 of 8 Small, multiple infarctions	Neuro sx+ Identified cause Embolic cause
Lauda et al,[44] 2015 (Germany)	2008–2013 213 Consecutive Aged 57–83 y Retrospective Systematic evaluation	TMVL: 68 BRAO: 44 CRAO: 101 + Neuro sx: 5	≤7 d of VL Standard stroke workup	DWI+ in 49 of 213 (23%) Same vascular territory as visual loss in 55% Small, multiple infarctions	Neuro sx+ CRAO > BRAO > TMVL Identified cause Embolic cause

Abbreviations: Neuro, neurological; sx, symptoms; TMVL, vascular transient monocular visual loss; VL, vision loss.

TREATMENT OF NONARTERITIC CENTRAL RETINAL ARTERY OCCLUSION OR BRANCH RETINAL ARTERY OCCLUSION

Treatment of CRAO can be divided into acute treatment (therapies directed at resolving the CRAO and improving visual outcome) and secondary prevention of subsequent ischemic events. No therapies have been shown to improve visual outcome following a nonarteritic CRAO beyond what is expected based on the natural history of CRAO. However, multiple interventions ranging from ocular massage and hyperventilation to IV and intra-arterial tissue plasminogen activator (tPA) have been attempted to restore ocular perfusion and, thus, improve visual outcome following a CRAO.[2,3,6,9,49] Theoretically, the sooner the retina is reperfused following an acute CRAO, the better the chance for improvement in visual function.[7,18,19] The ideal therapeutic window remains debated; but primate studies of arterial occlusions suggest that, similar to cerebral ischemia, any acute treatment would need to be administered within 3 hours of visual loss to prevent permanent retinal ischemia. Although it is possible that treatments administered within 6 to 12 hours of vision loss may prove beneficial, it is very unlikely that any treatment after 12 hours would have any effect, thereby limiting the value of many of the studies discussed later, in which treatment interventions were administered more than 12 to 24 hours after the onset of visual loss. However, because no acute treatment of CRAO has been shown to improve visual outcome, a larger emphasis should be placed on secondary prevention of systemic ischemic events (MI and cerebral infarction) following a CRAO, as systemic ischemia may prove more devastating than the CRAO itself.

CLASSIC OR CONVENTIONAL THERAPIES

Dislodging the Embolus

Ocular massage

Ocular massage is performed by compressing the globe with digital pressure over a closed eyelid for 10 to 20 minutes. The goal of ocular massage is to increase retinal artery perfusion and potentially dislodge a thrombus or embolus by causing retinal arteriolar dilatation and decreasing IOP.[6,13,50] However, the use of ocular massage, either alone or in combination with medications to reduce IOP, has not been shown to significantly alter the natural history of CRAO.[6,13,51]

Laser embolectomy

Physical dislodging of a visible embolus in CRAO by the use of a Nd:YAG laser application has been reported in a few cases.[52,53] Although in all cases, the investigators report improvement in retinal perfusion and visual function following the removal of the embolus, the procedure was complicated by vitreous hemorrhage in approximately 50% of patients and the formation of a false aneurysm of the CRA in one case.[52,53] The use of a ND:YAG laser in the treatment of CRAO is controversial and is not considered standard of care.

Increasing Retinal Artery Perfusion Pressure

Intraocular pressure–lowering medications

The use of IOP-lowering medications, either topical agents classically used for glaucoma or systemic medications (oral or IV acetazolamide or IV mannitol), have also been used in the acute management of CRAO to increase retinal arterial perfusion pressure.[13,54] Similar to the aforementioned interventions, there are no conclusive data to suggest that use of either topical or systemic IOP-lowering medications improve visual outcome following an acute CRAO.[13,55]

Anterior chamber paracentesis

Anterior chamber paracentesis (accomplished by inserting the needle of a small-gauge syringe through the limbal cornea into the anterior chamber and withdrawing a small amount of aqueous humor) causes a rapid decrease in the IOP, leading to dilatation of retinal arteries and increased retinal artery perfusion pressure.[17,56] Although a commonly used treatment of CRAO, anterior chamber paracentesis, similar to the effect of other IOP-lowering treatments, has not been shown to improve visual outcome in patients with CRAO.[49,51,56]

Vasodilatation

Hyperventilation or inhalation of carbogen

Inhalation of carbogen, a variable mixture of oxygen (eg, 95%) and carbon dioxide (CO_2) (eg, 5%), or hyperventilating into a brown bag increases the CO_2 concentration of the blood leading to a respiratory acidosis. An increased blood CO_2 concentration should prevent oxygen-induced vasoconstriction of retinal vasculature and cause retinal arteriolar dilatation, thereby increasing retinal perfusion and improving visual outcome following a CRAO.[56–59] However, the inhalation of carbogen or the use of hyperventilation does not produce any appreciable improvement in visual outcome compared with patients who received no acute intervention.[56]

Medications to induce vasodilation or increase erythrocyte flexibility

Systemic medications, such as sublingual isosorbide dinitrate and pentoxifylline, have also been used in the treatment of CRAO. Isosorbide dinitrate causes dilation of retinal vasculature and a mild decrease in IOP, increasing retinal arterial perfusion pressure. Similar to the effect of IOP-lowering medications, carbogen, and ocular massage, the use of isosorbide dinitrate has not been shown to improve visual outcome in CRAO.[13] Pentoxifylline is an oral medication that has been shown to increase red blood cell flexibility, reduce blood viscosity, and increase tissue perfusion.[60,61] In a small randomized controlled trial, pentoxifylline administration following a CRAO was shown to significantly increase CRA blood flow.[60] Because the effect of pentoxifylline on visual outcomes was not reported in these patients, there is no evidence in the literature to support its use in the acute treatment of CRAO.

Increasing Blood Oxygen Tension

Hyperbaric oxygen

Hyperbaric oxygen therapy is sometimes used in an acute CRAO to increase the oxygen tension leading to increased concentration of soluble oxygen in the blood, thereby increasing the relative amount of oxygen delivered to ischemic retinal tissue.[62,63] Hyperbaric oxygen therapy is used as a supportive measure until spontaneous reperfusion of the retina occurs or other modalities are used to restore retinal perfusion.[3] Although there have been case series suggesting improvement in visual function following hyperbaric oxygen therapy for CRAO, the improvement in visual function was not statistically significant compared with patients who did not receive hyperbaric oxygen therapy.[64,65] Specifically, in the study by Menzel-Severing and colleagues,[65] most patients who did not receive hyperbaric oxygen therapy had similar visual acuity at the 3-month follow-up visit compared with the patients who received hyperbaric oxygen treatment.

THROMBOLYSIS

Based on their use and efficacy in the treatment of acute cerebral ischemia, thrombolytics, such as urokinase, streptokinase, and, more recently, tPA, have been used in the treatment of acute CRAO. These agents convert plasminogen to plasmin and lead to dissolution of fibrin-based clots, which are thought to be the most common type of clot in CRAO.[6,8,9] Because there is no standard treatment regimen for the use of thrombolytics in CRAO, most clinicians base their use on established stroke protocols. Unfortunately, based on the current literature, including randomized controlled clinical trials, the use of thrombolytics has not been shown to reliably improve visual outcome in patients with a CRAO. Most of these studies administered thrombolysis more than 12 hours after visual loss, which may explain the low rate of vision improvement. In addition, the use of intra-arterial thrombolytics for CRAO was reported to have a high complication rate in the EAGLE trial; therefore, physicians must carefully consider the risks and benefits of thrombolysis in the management of acute CRAO on a case-by-case basis.

Intravenous or Intra-arterial Tissue Plasminogen Activator

Several retrospective reviews, case reports, and observational studies have suggested that tPA improved visual outcome in CRAO,[66–72] whereas other retrospective reviews and observational studies have reported no significant improvement in visual outcome in patients treated with tPA.[73–75]

For example, a retrospective analysis of 42 patients with an acute CRAO, defined as symptom onset of 15 hours or less, treated with conservative therapy alone or in combination with localized intra-arterial tPA, delivered into the origin of the ophthalmic artery in 30-mg aliquots up to a maximum of 20 mg, showed that there was a significant improvement in visual acuity in patients treated with conservative therapy and intra-arterial tPA.[66] Sixteen patients (76.2%) treated with intra-arterial tPA had an improvement in visual acuity of one or more lines compared with 7 patients (33.3%) treated with conservative therapy alone, suggesting that intra-arterial tPA is a viable treatment of an acute CRAO.[66]

The EAGLE trial,[76] a European multicenter, randomized controlled trial that compared the effect of intra-arterial tPA to conservative treatment (hemodilution, ocular massage, IOP-lowering medications, IV heparin, daily aspirin) on 82 patients with an acute CRAO, defined as symptom onset of 20 hours or less, did not show an improvement in visual acuity in the tPA cohort. Forty-two patients (51.2%) received localized intra-arterial thrombolysis into the ophthalmic artery or external carotid artery collaterals into the ophthalmic artery in predetermined increments of 15 mg, 30 mg, 45 mg, and a maximum dose of 50 mg of recombinant tPA.[76] No statistically significant improvement in visual acuity was found in patients treated with intra-arterial tPA compared with conservative treatment; 57.1% of patients in the thrombolysis group and 60.0% of patients in the conservative treatment group experienced 3 or more lines of improvement in visual acuity. However, 4.3% of patients in the conservative treatment group and 37.1% of patients in the thrombolysis group experienced adverse reactions, including intracranial hemorrhages, hemiparesis, headaches, dizziness, epistaxis, oral hemorrhage, and postprocedural hemorrhage. Because the study failed to show a significant improvement in visual acuity in patients treated with intra-arterial tPA compared with conservative treatment and there was an increased incidence of adverse events in the tPA group, the study was stopped prematurely at the first interim analysis.[76]

Similar to the results of the EAGLE trial, a placebo-controlled randomized trial studying the effect of IV tPA on visual outcome in patients with CRAO did not show a significant improvement in visual acuity in patients treated with IV tPA.[77] In 8 patients with an acute CRAO, defined as symptom onset of less than 24 hours, IV tPA was administered at a total dose of 0.9 mg/kg infused over 1 hour, with 10% of the total dose given in a bolus during the first minute of the infusion. Two of the 8 patients (25%) treated with IV tPA had an improvement in visual acuity of 3 or more lines compared with 0 of the 8 control patients, who received an IV saline infusion. Both of these patients received IV tPA within 6 hours of symptom onset. However, at the 1-month, 3-month, and 6-month evaluations, none of the patients treated with tPA had an improvement in visual acuity greater than their baseline presenting visual acuity, including the 2 patients who previously had improved visual acuity following IV tPA.[77] In addition, one patient in the IV tPA cohort developed an intracranial hemorrhage within 45 minutes of the tPA infusion.

The equivocal effectiveness of tPA in improving visual outcome in retrospective and observational studies of CRAO; the lack of improvement in visual outcome following administration of tPA in randomized controlled studies; the increased risk of adverse events associated with the administration of tPA; and the heterogeneity in study designs, including drug regimens, time to delivery of medication following CRAO, and study end points,[78] makes it extremely difficult to suggest therapeutic guidelines based on the available literature. Although there continues to be a trend in the literature suggesting that early intervention with tPA (less than 6 hours from symptom onset) is associated with improvement in visual outcome in CRAO,[69,77–79] further studies would be necessary to determine if there is indeed a significant improvement in visual outcome in patients with a CRAO treated with tPA either intravenously or intra-arterially within 6 hours of symptom onset. Unfortunately, multiple barriers exist to the design and completion of such studies, such as the rarity of CRAO and the delay in patient referral.

Although acute treatments have not been shown to improve visual outcomes in patients with CRAO, there is still hope for thrombolysis performed shortly after a CRAO. However, based on the currently available literature, the treatment of CRAO should be focused on identifying a concomitant acute cerebral infarction, which is a medical emergency; optimization of all cardiovascular risk factors; and a thorough investigation for undiagnosed cardiovascular risk factors, with the ultimate goal being prevention of subsequent ischemic events, such as an acute MI, vascular death, and acute cerebral ischemia. Therefore, optimal management of these patients requires collaboration between ophthalmologists and stroke neurologists, the former to make the initial diagnosis and monitor for any subsequent retinal ischemic events and for secondary ocular complications, such as neovascularization, and the latter to perform the acute workup, optimize known cardiovascular risk factors, assess for undiagnosed cardiovascular risk factors, and monitor for any evidence of further systemic ischemic events.

REFERENCES

1. Graefes A. Ueber Embolie der Arteria centralis retinae als Ursache plotzlicher Erblindung. Arch Ophthalmol 1859;5:136–57.
2. Biousse V, Newman N. Retinal and optic nerve ischemia. Continuum (Minneap Minn) 2014;20:838–56.
3. Cugati S, Varma DD, Chen CS, et al. Treatment options for central retinal artery occlusion. Curr Treat Options Neurol 2013;15:63–77.
4. Lorentzen SE. Incidence of cilioretinal arteries. Acta Ophthalmol (Copenh) 1970; 48:518–24.
5. Hayreh SS. Ocular vascular occlusive disorders: natural history of visual outcome. Prog Retin Eye Res 2014;41:1–25.
6. Chen CS, Lee AW. Management of acute central retinal artery occlusion. Nat Clin Pract Neurol 2008;4:376–83.

7. Hayreh SS, Zimmerman MB. Central retinal artery occlusion: visual outcome. Am J Ophthalmol 2005;140:376–91.
8. Rudkin AK, Lee AW, Chen CS. Vascular risk factors for central retinal artery occlusion. Eye (Lond) 2010;24:678–81.
9. Varma DD, Cugati S, Lee AW, et al. A review of central retinal artery occlusion: clinical presentation and management. Eye (Lond) 2013;27:688–97.
10. Biousse V. Acute retinal arterial ischemia: an emergency often ignored. Am J Ophthalmol 2014;157:1119–21.
11. Leavitt JA, Larson TA, Hodge DO, et al. The incidence of central retinal artery occlusion in Olmsted County, Minnesota. Am J Ophthalmol 2011;152:820–3.e2.
12. Park SJ, Choi NK, Seo KH, et al. Nationwide incidence of clinically diagnosed central retinal artery occlusion in Korea, 2008 to 2011. Ophthalmology 2014; 121:1933–8.
13. Rumelt S, Dorenboim Y, Rehany U. Aggressive systematic treatment for central retinal artery occlusion. Am J Ophthalmol 1999;128:733–8.
14. Hayreh SS, Podhajsky PA, Zimmerman MB. Retinal artery occlusion: associated systemic and ophthalmic abnormalities. Ophthalmology 2009;116:1928–36.
15. Hayreh SS, Zimmerman MB. Fundus changes in central retinal artery occlusion. Retina 2007;27:276–89.
16. Shinoda K, Yamada K, Matsumoto CS, et al. Changes in retinal thickness are correlated with alterations of electroretinogram in eyes with central retinal artery occlusion. Graefes Arch Clin Exp Ophthalmol 2008;246:949–54.
17. Beatty S, Au Eong KG. Acute occlusion of the retinal arteries: current concepts and recent advances in diagnosis and management. J Accid Emerg Med 2000;17:324–9.
18. Hayreh SS, Jonas JB. Optic disk and retinal nerve fiber layer damage after transient central retinal artery occlusion: an experimental study in rhesus monkeys. Am J Ophthalmol 2000;129:786–95.
19. Hayreh SS, Zimmerman MB, Kimura A, et al. Central retinal artery occlusion. Retinal survival time. Exp Eye Res 2004;78:723–36.
20. Hayreh SS. Acute retinal arterial occlusive disorders. Prog Retin Eye Res 2011; 30:359–94.
21. Schmidt D, Hetzel A, Geibel-Zehender A, et al. Systemic diseases in non-inflammatory branch and central retinal artery occlusion–an overview of 416 patients. Eur J Med Res 2007;12:595–603.
22. Callizo J, Feltgen N, Pantenburg S, et al, European Assessment Group for Lysis in the Eye. Cardiovascular risk factors in central retinal artery occlusion: results of a prospective and standardized medical examination. Ophthalmology 2015;122: 1881–8.
23. Douglas DJ, Schuler JJ, Buchbinder D, et al. The association of central retinal artery occlusion and extracranial carotid artery disease. Ann Surg 1988;208:85–90.
24. Klein R, Klein BE, Moss SE, et al. Retinal emboli and cardiovascular disease: the Beaver Dam Eye Study. Arch Ophthalmol 2003;121:1446–51.
25. Biousse V, Touboul PJ, D'Anglejan-Chatillon J, et al. Ophthalmologic manifestations of internal carotid artery dissection. Am J Ophthalmol 1998;126:565–77.
26. Patel M, Shah G, Davies JB, et al. Re-evaluating our perspective on retinal artery occlusion from carotid dissection: a report of three cases and review of the literature. Ophthalmic Surg Lasers Imaging Retina 2013;44:555–60.
27. Brown GC, Magargal LE, Shields JA, et al. Retinal arterial obstruction in children and young adults. Ophthalmology 1981;88:18–25.

28. Bruno A, Jones WL, Austin JK, et al. Vascular outcome in men with asymptomatic retinal cholesterol emboli. A cohort study. Ann Intern Med 1995;122:249–53.
29. Chang SH, Miller NR. The incidence of vision loss due to perioperative ischemic optic neuropathy associated with spine surgery: the Johns Hopkins Hospital Experience. Spine (Phila Pa 1976) 2005;30:1299–302.
30. Sys J, Michielsen J, Mertens E, et al. Central retinal artery occlusion after spinal surgery. Eur Spine J 1996;5:74–5.
31. Park SW, Woo SJ, Park KH, et al. Iatrogenic retinal artery occlusion caused by cosmetic facial filler injections. Am J Ophthalmol 2012;154:653–62.e1.
32. Hankey GJ, Slattery JM, Warlow CP. Prognosis and prognostic factors of retinal infarction: a prospective cohort study. BMJ 1991;302:499–504.
33. Helenius J, Arsava EM, Goldstein JN, et al. Concurrent acute brain infarcts in patients with monocular visual loss. Ann Neurol 2012;72:286–93.
34. Park SJ, Choi NK, Yang BR, et al. Risk and risk periods for stroke and acute myocardial infarction in patients with central retinal artery occlusion. Ophthalmology 2015;122:2336–43.e2.
35. Rim TH, Han J, Choi YS, et al. Retinal artery occlusion and the risk of stroke development: twelve-year nationwide cohort study. Stroke 2016;47:376–82.
36. Vu HT, Keeffe JE, Mccarty CA, et al. Impact of unilateral and bilateral vision loss on quality of life. Br J Ophthalmol 2005;89:360–3.
37. Rudkin AK, Lee AW, Chen CS. Ocular neovascularization following central retinal artery occlusion: prevalence and timing of onset. Eur J Ophthalmol 2010;20:1042–6.
38. Klein R, Klein BE, Jensen SC, et al. Retinal emboli and stroke: the Beaver Dam Eye Study. Arch Ophthalmol 1999;117:1063–8.
39. Wang JJ, Cugati S, Knudtson MD, et al. Retinal arteriolar emboli and long-term mortality: pooled data analysis from two older populations. Stroke 2006;37:1833–6.
40. Chang YS, Jan RL, Weng SF, et al. Retinal artery occlusion and the 3-year risk of stroke in Taiwan: a nationwide population-based study. Am J Ophthalmol 2012;154:645–52.e1.
41. Sacco RL, Kasner SE, Broderick JP, et al, American Heart Association Stroke Council, Council on Cardiovascular Surgery and Anesthesia, Council on Cardiovascular Radiology and Intervention, Council on Cardiovascular and Stroke Nursing, Council on Epidemiology and Prevention, Council on Peripheral Vascular Disease, Council on Nutrition, Physical Activity and Metabolism. An updated definition of stroke for the 21st century: a statement for healthcare professionals from the American Heart Association/American Stroke Association. Stroke 2013;44:2064–89.
42. Atkins EJ, Bruce BB, Newman NJ, et al. Translation of clinical studies to clinical practice: survey on the treatment of central retinal artery occlusion. Am J Ophthalmol 2009;148:172–3.
43. Biousse V, Trobe JD. Transient monocular visual loss. Am J Ophthalmol 2005;140:717–21.
44. Lauda F, Neugebauer H, Reiber L, et al. Acute silent brain infarction in monocular visual loss of ischemic origin. Cerebrovasc Dis 2015;40:151–6.
45. Lee J, Kim SW, Lee SC, et al. Co-occurrence of acute retinal artery occlusion and acute ischemic stroke: diffusion-weighted magnetic resonance imaging study. Am J Ophthalmol 2014;157:1231–8.
46. Greven CM, Slusher MM, Weaver RG. Retinal arterial occlusions in young adults. Am J Ophthalmol 1995;120:776–83.

47. Bossert M, Prati C, Balblanc JC, et al. Aortic involvement in giant cell arteritis: current data. Joint Bone Spine 2011;78:246–51.
48. Dasgupta B, Borg FA, Hassan N, et al. BSR and BHPR guidelines for the management of giant cell arteritis. Rheumatology (Oxford) 2010;49:1594–7.
49. Fraser SG, Adams W. Interventions for acute non-arteritic central retinal artery occlusion. Cochrane Database Syst Rev 2009;(1):CD001989.
50. Augsburger JJ, Magargal LE. Visual prognosis following treatment of acute central retinal artery obstruction. Br J Ophthalmol 1980;64:913–7.
51. Rudkin AK, Lee AW, Aldrich E, et al. Clinical characteristics and outcome of current standard management of central retinal artery occlusion. Clin Exp Ophthalmol 2010;38:496–501.
52. Opremcak E, Rehmar AJ, Ridenour CD, et al. Restoration of retinal blood flow via translumenal Nd:YAG embolysis/embolectomy (TYL/E) for central and branch retinal artery occlusion. Retina 2008;28:226–35.
53. Reynard M, Hanscom TA. Neodymium:yttrium-aluminum-garnet laser arteriotomy with embolectomy for central retinal artery occlusion. Am J Ophthalmol 2004;137:196–8.
54. Rassam SM, Patel V, Kohner EM. The effect of acetazolamide on the retinal circulation. Eye (Lond) 1993;7(Pt 5):697–702.
55. Landa E, Rehany U, Rumelt S. Visual functions following recovery from nonarteritic central retinal artery occlusion. Ophthalmic Surg Lasers Imaging 2004;35:103–8.
56. Atebara NH, Brown GC, Cater J. Efficacy of anterior chamber paracentesis and carbogen in treating acute nonarteritic central retinal artery occlusion. Ophthalmology 1995;102:2029–34 [discussion: 2034–5].
57. Arend O, Harris A, Martin BJ, et al. Retinal blood velocities during carbogen breathing using scanning laser ophthalmoscopy. Acta Ophthalmol (Copenh) 1994;72:332–6.
58. Deutsch TA, Read JS, Ernest JT, et al. Effects of oxygen and carbon dioxide on the retinal vasculature in humans. Arch Ophthalmol 1983;101:1278–80.
59. Harino S, Grunwald JE, Petrig BJ, et al. Rebreathing into a bag increases human retinal macular blood velocity. Br J Ophthalmol 1995;79:380–3.
60. Incandela L, Cesarone MR, Belcaro G, et al. Treatment of vascular retinal disease with pentoxifylline: a controlled, randomized trial. Angiology 2002;53(Suppl 1):S31–4.
61. Iwafune Y, Yoshimoto H. Clinical use of pentoxifylline in haemorrhagic disorders of the retina. Pharmatherapeutica 1980;2:429–38.
62. Anderson B Jr, Saltzman HA, Heyman A. The effects of hyperbaric oxygenation on retinal arterial occlusion. Arch Ophthalmol 1965;73:315–9.
63. Beiran I, Goldenberg I, Adir Y, et al. Early hyperbaric oxygen therapy for retinal artery occlusion. Eur J Ophthalmol 2001;11:345–50.
64. Cope A, Eggert JV, O'Brien E. Retinal artery occlusion: visual outcome after treatment with hyperbaric oxygen. Diving Hyperb Med 2011;41:135–8.
65. Menzel-Severing J, Siekmann U, Weinberger A, et al. Early hyperbaric oxygen treatment for nonarteritic central retinal artery obstruction. Am J Ophthalmol 2012;153:454–9.e2.
66. Aldrich EM, Lee AW, Chen CS, et al. Local intraarterial fibrinolysis administered in aliquots for the treatment of central retinal artery occlusion: the Johns Hopkins Hospital experience. Stroke 2008;39:1746–50.

67. Arnold M, Koerner U, Remonda L, et al. Comparison of intra-arterial thrombolysis with conventional treatment in patients with acute central retinal artery occlusion. J Neurol Neurosurg Psychiatry 2005;76:196–9.
68. Biousse V, Calvetti O, Bruce BB, et al. Thrombolysis for central retinal artery occlusion. J Neuroophthalmol 2007;27:215–30.
69. Hattenbach LO, Kuhli-Hattenbach C, Scharrer I, et al. Intravenous thrombolysis with low-dose recombinant tissue plasminogen activator in central retinal artery occlusion. Am J Ophthalmol 2008;146:700–6.
70. Hwang G, Woo SJ, Jung C, et al. Intra-arterial thrombolysis for central retinal artery occlusion: two cases report. J Korean Med Sci 2010;25:974–9.
71. Noble J, Weizblit N, Baerlocher MO, et al. Intra-arterial thrombolysis for central retinal artery occlusion: a systematic review. Br J Ophthalmol 2008;92:588–93.
72. Nowak RJ, Amin H, Robeson K, et al. Acute central retinal artery occlusion treated with intravenous recombinant tissue plasminogen activator. J Stroke Cerebrovasc Dis 2012;21:913.e5-8.
73. Agarwal N, Gala NB, Karimi RJ, et al. Current endovascular treatment options for central retinal arterial occlusion: a review. Neurosurg Focus 2014;36:E7.
74. Ahn SJ, Kim JM, Hong JH, et al. Efficacy and safety of intra-arterial thrombolysis in central retinal artery occlusion. Invest Ophthalmol Vis Sci 2013;54:7746–55.
75. Pettersen JA, Hill MD, Demchuk AM, et al. Intra-arterial thrombolysis for retinal artery occlusion: the Calgary experience. Can J Neurol Sci 2005;32:507–11.
76. Schumacher M, Schmidt D, Jurklies B, et al, EAGLE-Study Group. Central retinal artery occlusion: local intra-arterial fibrinolysis versus conservative treatment, a multicenter randomized trial. Ophthalmology 2010;117:1367–75.e1.
77. Chen CS, Lee AW, Campbell B, et al. Efficacy of intravenous tissue-type plasminogen activator in central retinal artery occlusion: report from a randomized, controlled trial. Stroke 2011;42:2229–34.
78. Biousse V. Thrombolysis for acute central retinal artery occlusion: is it time? Am J Ophthalmol 2008;146:631–4.
79. Egan RA, Van Stavern R. Should patients with acute central retinal artery occlusion be treated with intra-arterial t-PA? J Neuroophthalmol 2015;35:205–9.

Imaging of Oculomotor (Third) Cranial Nerve Palsy

Michael S. Vaphiades, DO[a,b,c,*], Glenn H. Roberson, MD[d]

KEYWORDS

- Magnetic resonance angiography (MRA)
- Computed tomography angiography (CTA)
- Intraarterial digital subtraction angiography (DSA)

KEY POINTS

- In clinical practice, most patients presenting with an oculomotor (third) cranial nerve palsy undergo some form of neuroimaging.
- A significant number of patients with a ruptured intracranial aneurysm resulting in subarachnoid hemorrhage (SAH) have an oculomotor palsy before rupture.
- Digital subtraction angiography (DSA) remains the gold standard study for imaging cerebral aneurysms, including those producing an oculomotor palsy.
- Computed tomography angiography (CTA) has supplanted DSA in many cases as the initial imaging study used to detect intracranial aneurysms.
- MR angiography remains a powerful alternative or complementary study to DSA and CTA for visualization of intracranial aneurysms, especially when there are artifacts or contraindications to these studies.

INTRODUCTION

In the management of a patient with presumed oculomotor cranial nerve palsy owing to aneurysmal compression, there is often debate on which initial mode of neuroimaging should be ordered: MR angiography (MRA), computed tomography angiography (CTA), or intraarterial digital subtraction angiography (DSA).[1] Clinically, compressive

This work was supported in part by an unrestricted grant from the Research to Prevent Blindness, Inc. New York, New York.
There are no commercial or financial conflicts of interest and any funding sources by either author.
[a] Department of Ophthalmology, University of Alabama at Birmingham, Suite 601, 700 South 18th Street, Birmingham, AL 35233, USA; [b] Department of Neurology, University of Alabama at Birmingham, 1720 2nd Avenue S, Birmingham, AL 35233, USA; [c] Department of Neurosurgery, University of Alabama at Birmingham, 1720 2nd Avenue S, Birmingham, AL 35233, USA; [d] Department of Radiology, University of Alabama at Birmingham, JT N420, 619 19th Street South, Birmingham, AL 35249-6830, USA
* Corresponding author. Department of Ophthalmology, University of Alabama at Birmingham, Suite 601, 700 South 18th Street, Birmingham, AL 35233.
E-mail address: vaph@uab.edu

Neurol Clin 35 (2017) 101–113
http://dx.doi.org/10.1016/j.ncl.2016.08.009 neurologic.theclinics.com

lesions of the oculomotor nerve owing to aneurysm often produce ptosis, a fixed, dilated ipsilateral pupil and a specific pattern of oculomotor nerve-related ophthalmoplegia (ie, the eye is "down and out," with complete ptosis). There should be intact abduction and evidence of incyclotorsion, indicating intact abducens and trochlear cranial nerves, respectively. In contrast, oculomotor cranial nerve palsy from an ischemic mononeuropathy such as diabetes or hypertension usually demonstrates little or no anisocoria and the pupil is usually reactive in the setting of complete ptosis and ophthalmoplegia. There are important amendments to these guidelines however:

1. Oculomotor cranial nerve palsy owing to an aneurysm at or near the junction of the internal carotid and posterior communicating arteries may initially demonstrate normal pupillary size and reactivity in up to 14% of patients (especially with partial somatic involvement), but pupillary involvement may develop in the ensuing 7 to 10 days.[2,3]
2. To be judged "pupil-sparing" third cranial nerve palsy, the isocoric and reactive pupil must be seen in a setting of complete ptosis and complete involvement of the muscles innervated by the oculomotor nerve.[3,4] If there is not complete ptosis and the correct pattern and severity of oculomotor nerve related ophthalmoplegia then "all bets are off."
3. In addition, ischemic oculomotor cranial nerve palsies have been reported to be "pupillary involving" in up to 32% of cases,[4] and the associated anisocoria may be as great as 2.5 mm.[5]
4. Pain may be present with both compressive and ischemic causes and therefore not very helpful in distinguishing between these 2 entities.[6]

In clinical practice, most patients presenting with oculomotor cranial nerve palsy, either pupil involving or sparing, undergo some form of neuroimaging study because the risk of missing a posterior communicating artery aneurysm is very high.

INTRACRANIAL ANEURYSMS

Up to 90% of intracranial aneurysms occur in the region of the circle of Willis.[7] The typical clinical presentation of SAH is severe headache, loss of consciousness, stiff neck, and nausea, and this entity may ultimately result in coma or death.[8] Rupture of an intracranial aneurysm with SAH has a mortality of up to 50%.[9] The overall frequency of intracranial aneurysms in the general population is approximately 5%, with a rupture rate for posterior communicating artery aneurysm being higher than anterior circulation aneurysms, at any sizes.[10] Studies have shown a risk of rupture of 0.52% for aneurysms 7 to 12 mm in diameter of the anterior circulation and 2.9% for aneurysms located in posterior circulation in same size category.[11] One study suggested that the critical size for aneurysm rupture ranges from 4 to 10 mm.[9] Still another calculated the rupture rate for unruptured intracranial aneurysms of less than 10 mm in diameter is 0.05% per year.[10] In patients with unruptured intracranial aneurysms of less than 7 mm in diameter who have not had a previous SAH, the rupture rate is about 0.1% per year[11] and for aneurysms greater than 10 mm it approaches 1% per year.[10] If the aneurysm is greater than 25 mm in diameter (giant aneurysm), the rupture rate is 6% in the first year.[10] Many factors, including site, size, and group-specific risks, are involved in management of these patients with unruptured intracranial aneurysms.[11] The smallest posterior communicating artery aneurysm reported to presumably cause a third nerve palsy is 3 mm,[12,13] yet most reports have maintained that a posterior communicating artery aneurysm needs to be at least 4 mm to cause a compressive third nerve palsy.[12] Thus, noninvasive tests like contrast-enhanced MRA and CTA are vital to the detection and management of unruptured intracranial aneurysms. These imaging studies are important alternatives to DSA because of complications of DSA discussed elsewhere in this paper.[14–16] Aneurysms at or near the junction of the internal carotid artery and posterior communicating artery are a common cause of an isolated third nerve palsy, yet other locations like basilar tip, cavernous sinus, or internal carotid artery (giant aneurysm) may also cause a third cranial nerve palsy. However, in this paper, we use posterior communicating artery aneurysm to refer to all aneurysms at or near this location because they are more likely to present with an isolated third nerve palsy compared with other aneurysm locations.[16]

DIGITAL SUBTRACTION ANGIOGRAPHY

DSA is also known as conventional angiography. This technique uses fluoroscopy and iodine-based intravascular contrast material. DSA "subtracts out" images of structures other than blood vessels such as bone, thus making the blood vessels more visible. The intracranial circulation is accessed using a catheter via the femoral artery. Individual great vessels are then identified and contrast is infused. DSA is generally associated with a 1% to 2% risk of complications, including stroke.[15,16] Therefore, this risk must be considered in the context of the potential benefits. DSA remains the definitive or "gold standard" test for imaging the intracranial and extracranial blood vessels, and particularly for detecting cerebral aneurysms. Because of the risk of potential morbidity, DSA studies have largely been replaced by less invasive techniques requiring no arterial catheter such as 3-dimensional (3D) CTA and MRA.[15,17] In 2010, Thiex and colleagues[18] evaluated 1715 consecutive patients undergoing DSA and assessed them retrospectively for stroke or transient ischemic attack presumably from the procedure. In 40 of the patients, diffusion-weighted MRI study had been serendipitously performed within the first 30 days after DSA. Two patients had punctate areas of restricted diffusion in territories that had been explored angiographically. No stroke or permanent neurologic deficit was seen in any of the 1715 patients. One patient experienced a transient ischemic attack. Nonneurologic complications without long-term sequelae occurred in 9 patients. So at their institution, the risk for neurologic complications related to DSA was less than 1%. DSA is superior to CTA and MRA in that it can detect aneurysms smaller than 3 mm in diameter.[19] However, is an aneurysm that small capable of causing a compressive third cranial nerve palsy? Again, the smallest posterior communicating artery aneurysm reported to cause a third nerve palsy is 3 mm,[12,13] with most being at least 4 mm in size.[12]

COMPUTED TOMOGRAPHY ANGIOGRAPHY

In neuroimaging, high spatial resolution resolves 2 linear structures of the same density in close proximity and high contrast resolution resolves 2 complex shapes of similar density in close proximity. High spatial resolution reduces contrast resolution. CT and MRI have low spatial resolution but much greater contrast resolution, whereas DSA is just the opposite, with the best spatial resolution.[20] Like DSA, in CTA this objective is met by the injection of contrast material intravascularly.[20] Also like DSA, the contrast is iodine based and ionizing radiation is used. However, because the contrast material is injected into an antecubital vein (intravenous) rather than the femoral artery (intraarterial DSA), CTA is associated with less morbidity. The intravenous bolus of contrast material is followed by high-speed spiral CT scanning; in fact, the patient is moved through the scanner during 1 breath hold.[17] This x-ray source circumnavigates the patient's head and acquires images that are transformed mathematically and collated such that 2 types of 3D displays are generated: shaded surface display

(**Fig. 1**) and maximum intensity projection (**Fig. 2**).[17,20] Shaded surface display shows surface anatomy in a 3D-type view (see **Fig. 1**). Color also helps create a "true life image." Maximum intensity projection shows only the blood vessels, without color, and looks more like an MRA source image than a shaded surface display image. Both types of images can be rotated in space and, with ever evolving multidetector scanners, the time to produce these complex images has lessened. Despite the complexity and beauty of these images, cranial CT without contrast is the preferred initial diagnostic study in patients with suspected SAH because acute blood looks hyperdense on the scan, often filling the cisterns and sulci; this scan may also display the pattern and site of hemorrhage if multiple aneurysms are present (**Figs. 3** and **4**).[7,16] The sensitivity of unenhanced CT scanning in the detection of SAH within the first 48 hours approaches 95%.[7] The sensitivity of CT scanning in the detection of SAH is close to that of lumbar puncture.[7,16] Once the SAH is identified, immediate CTA (patient already in the gantry) is obtained to define the aneurysm[7] (see **Fig. 1**). Hence, if a CTA shows the intracranial aneurysm, a DSA is usually not required for surgery. If the CTA is negative, then the next step is usually DSA.[7,16] CTA has good correlation with DSA with exquisite delineation of intracranial anatomy (**Fig. 5**). In 1 study, CTA detected intracranial aneurysms as small as 3 mm in size.[21] A recent metaanalysis of 45 studies compared CTA with DSA and/or intraoperative findings in patients suspected of having cerebral aneurysms. They found that the diagnostic accuracy of CTA with 16- or 64-row multidetector was significantly higher than that of single-detector CT, especially in detecting small aneurysms of 4 mm or less in diameter. They concluded that CTA may one day selectively replace DSA in patients suspected of having a cerebral aneurysm when using a multidetector unit.[22] In fact, 1 author went further and stated that the sensitivity of CTA for the detection of cerebral aneurysms less than or equal to 5 mm is greater than that of DSA, with equal specificity and high interoperator reliability.[19] Because CTA is now widely used as a routine primary tool in the diagnosis of intracranial aneurysms, there is concern that the radiation dose has been increasing with potential

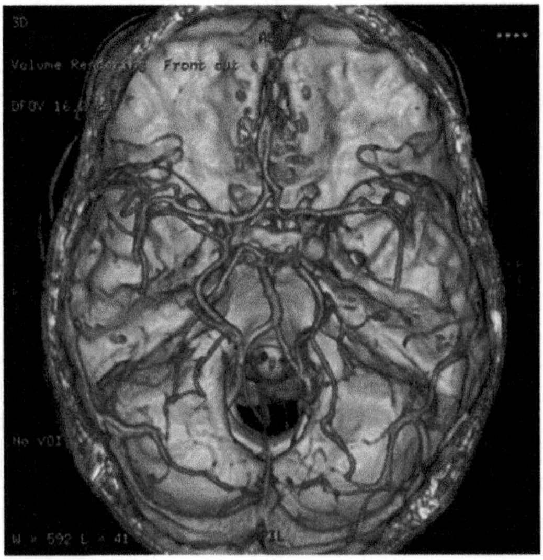

Fig. 1. Computed tomography angiography: 3-dimensional color-rendered angiogram. Note the projection is from above, and the right posterior communicating aneurysm is on the right side of the scan.

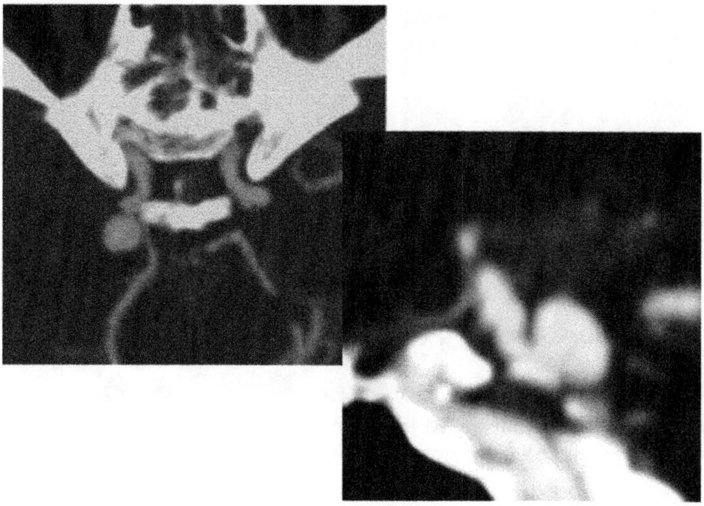

Fig. 2. Computed tomography angiography. Axial (*left*) maximal image projection and oblique sagittal (*right*) views of the right posterior communicating aneurysm. Note relation to cavernous sinus and sella.

harm to the brain.[23,24] With this in mind, 294 consecutive patients with spontaneous SAH was studied prospectively and assigned randomly to either conventional voltage CTA or low voltage CTA and analyzed for quality, radiation dose, and accuracy of the scan. The authors found no significant differences in sensitivity, specificity, and accuracy between the conventional voltage CTA and low voltage CTA groups and concluded that low voltage CTA should be recommended as a routine scanning method for the detection of aneurysms because of the lower radiation dose.[23] As revolutionary as CTA has become, there are disadvantages other than radiation dose; for example, an aneurysm may be obscured by boney artifact near the skull base or

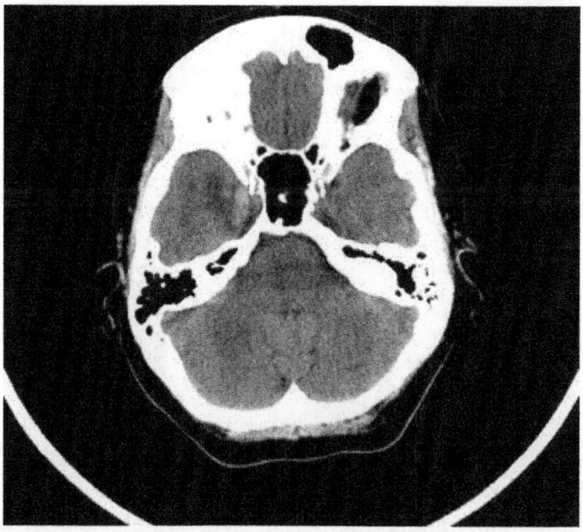

Fig. 3. Axial unenhanced computed tomography scan showing slight hemorrhage in the right paracavernous region.

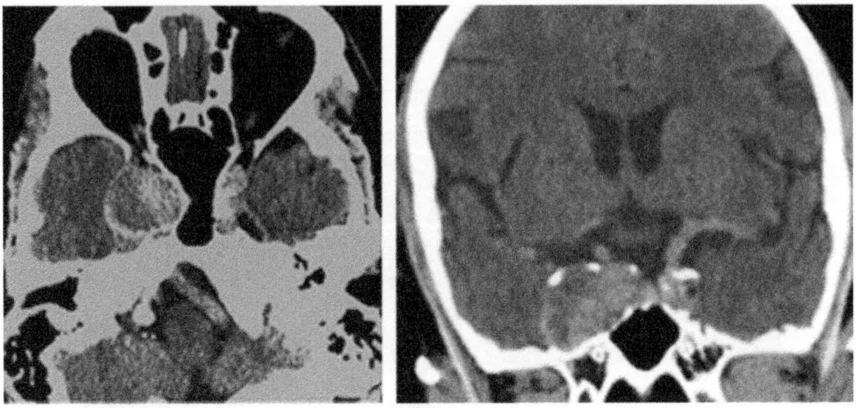

Fig. 4. Axial (*left*) and coronal (*right*) unenhanced computed tomography scans showing calcification in the wall of a giant right posterior communicating artery aneurysm.

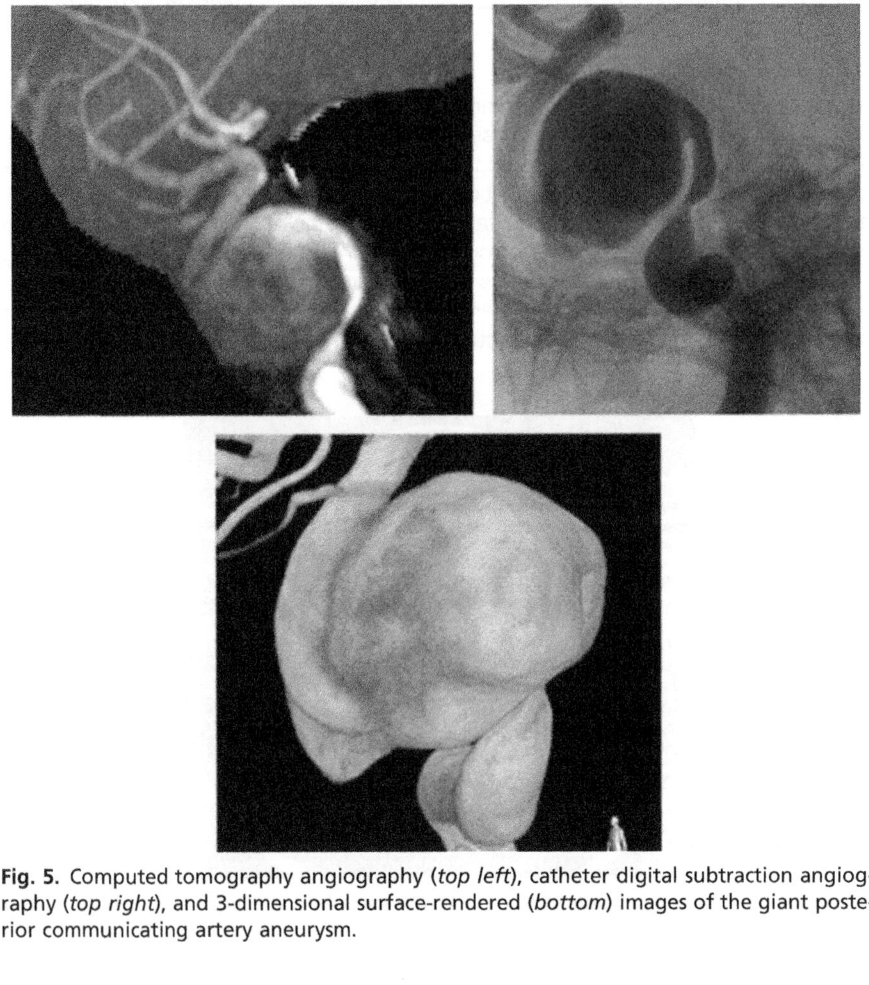

Fig. 5. Computed tomography angiography (*top left*), catheter digital subtraction angiography (*top right*), and 3-dimensional surface-rendered (*bottom*) images of the giant posterior communicating artery aneurysm.

cavernous sinus where MRA may be superior.[14,15] The advantages of CTA over MRA include shorter scanning times and better resolution of images. CTA can also be used safely in patients with implanted metal objects (such as shrapnel, pacemakers, and older aneurysm clips), which preclude the use of MRI, and is superior to MRI when claustrophobia makes MRI scanning impractical.

MR ANGIOGRAPHY

MRA does not use ionizing radiation or iodinated contrast material, unlike DSA and CTA. In terms of radiation exposure from CT, 1 study estimated that of approximately 600,000 abdominal and head CT examinations performed annually in the United States in children less than 15 years of age, 500 of these individuals might ultimately die from cancer attributable to the CT radiation.[25] Granted, the incidence of SAH increases with age (mean age of approximately 50 years), this pediatric radiation data is also important for young adults, especially given that the US population is living longer. Another advantage of MRA is the flexibility of the display (images of blood vessels can be rotated and viewed from different angles; **Fig. 6**) as well as use in renal failure patients where nephrogenic systemic fibrosis (a rare disorder that occurs in patients with reduced renal function after MRI gadolinium administration) is a concern.[7] There are 3 types of MRA techniques: 3D time of flight (TOF; **Figs. 7** and **8**), 2-dimensional (2D) TOF (**Fig. 9**), and contrast-enhanced MRA (**Figs. 10** and **11**).[26] The first 2 techniques do not require gadolinium, but depend on directional blood flow to generate images.[27] Frequently, all 3 techniques are used to generate MRA images.[27,28] Contrast-enhanced MRA is used to image both the head and neck vasculature, particularly the aortic arch and great neck vessels. Two-dimensional TOF is used to image the carotid arteries and 3D TOF is used to image the intracranial vessels. To generate a TOF image, data must be obtained from flow characteristics of blood and a saturation pulse is used to subtract out the veins. Owing to the physiology of blood flow, blood vessel diameter may seem to be smaller than it actually is, thereby leading to the potential for MRA to "overcall" the degree of vascular stenosis (as in the assessment of the carotid arteries). In this setting, carotid Doppler ultrasonography and DSA may provide more accurate measurements of the degree of carotid stenosis.

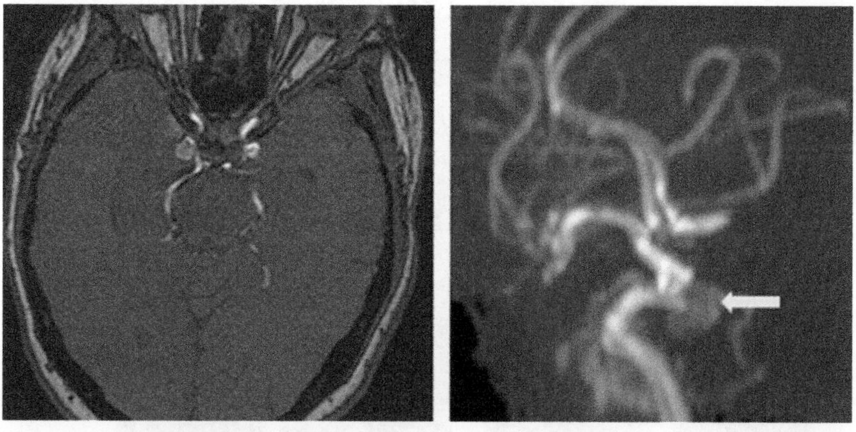

Fig. 6. Three-dimensional (3D) MR angiography. Axial source image (maximal image projection) (*left*) and sagittal 3D time of flight image (*right*) showing a partially thrombosed posterior communicating artery aneurysm (*arrow*).

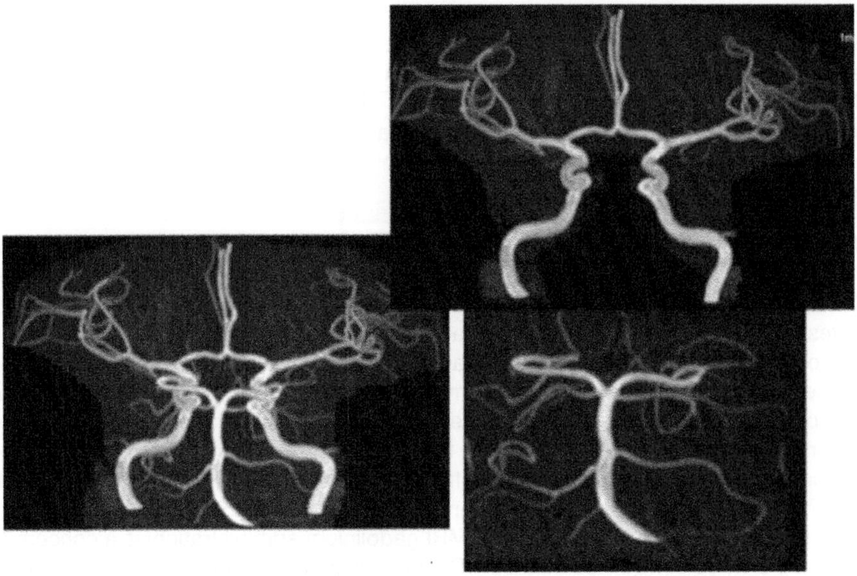

Fig. 7. Three-dimensional time of flight MR angiography. Image signal intensity is proportional to flow. Vascular compartments have been manually separated.

In addition, 1 very important disadvantage of MRA is the underestimation of intracranial aneurysm size or failure to detect aneurysms all together, even in the clinical setting or oculomotor cranial nerve palsy.[15,29] In fact, patients with oculomotor cranial nerve palsy from posterior communicating artery aneurysms measuring up to 7 mm

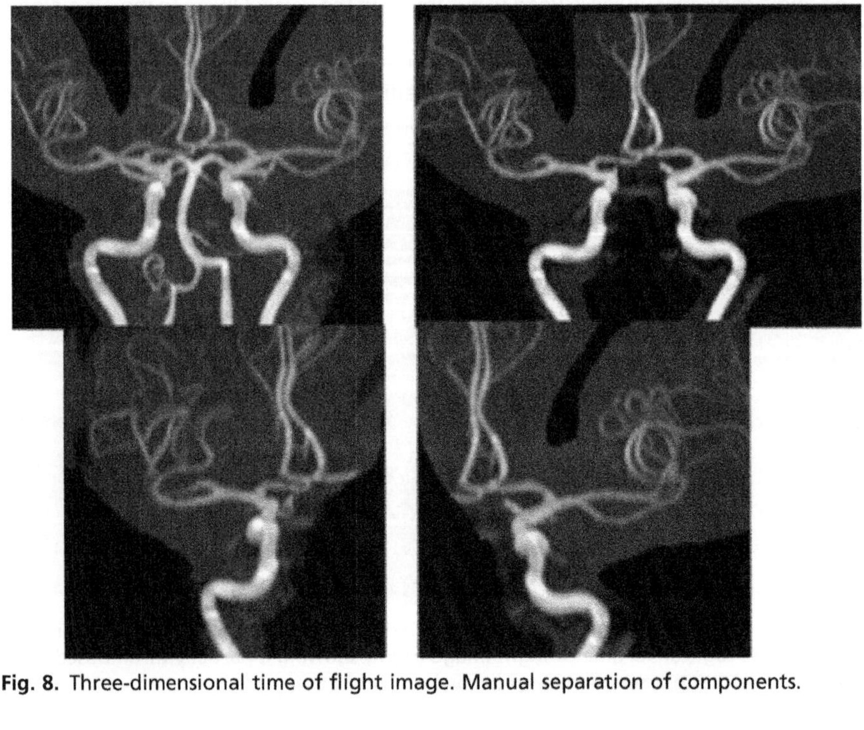

Fig. 8. Three-dimensional time of flight image. Manual separation of components.

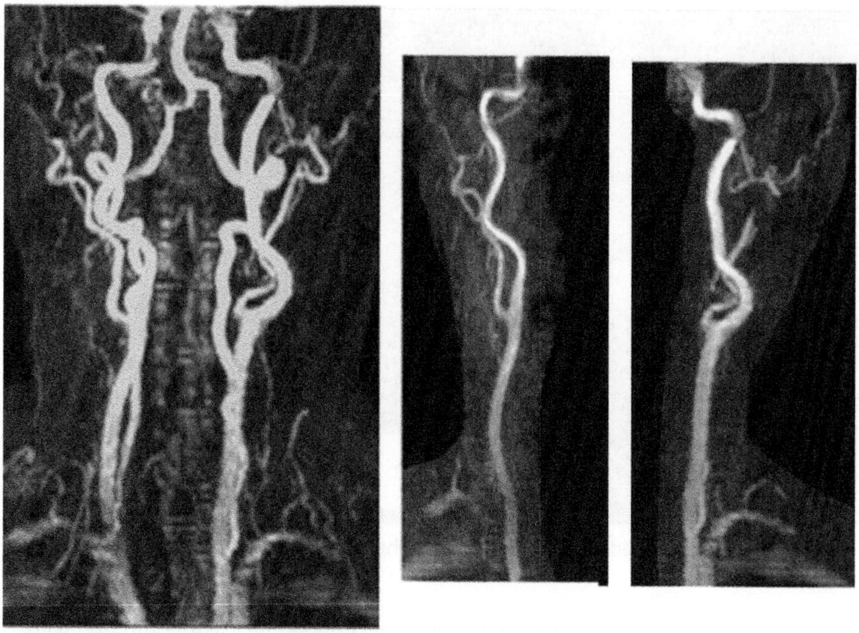

Fig. 9. Two-dimensional time of flight MR angiography. Signal is proportional to flow and is directionally encoded; only antegrade flow is displayed.

have been missed by MRA.[1] One study concluded that only a 2-mm aneurysm seen on catheter-based angiography was missed by MRA, yet this is facility dependent and magnet dependent.[30] The authors also indicated that in their study, symptomatic aneurysms were equal or greater than 4 mm in size.[30] One study examined 47 patients

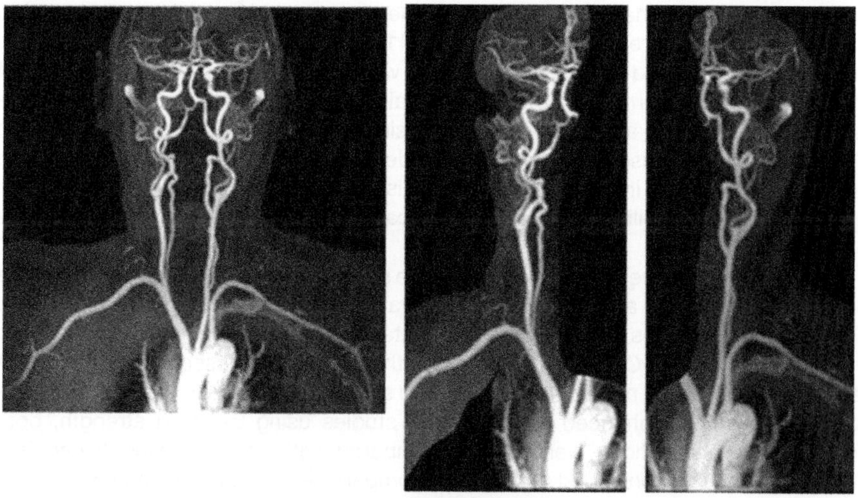

Fig. 10. Contrast-enhanced MR angiography with intravenous injection of Gadolinium. Vascular compartments manually separated. Signal intensity is very strong with excellent detail.

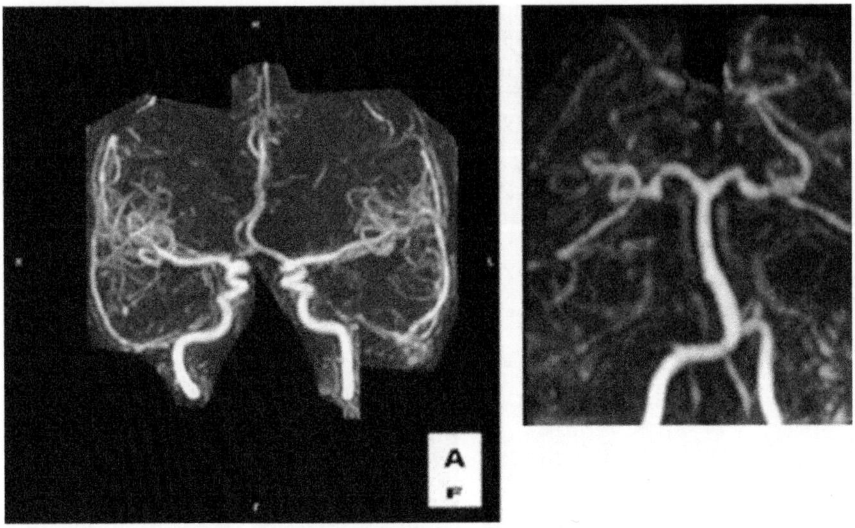

Fig. 11. Contrast-enhanced MR angiography of the head only.

who had saccular or giant intracranial aneurysms imaged by MRA compared with 19 patients imaged with DSA. The remaining 28 patients, in whom no aneurysm was found, served as a control group. The study concluded that MRA can define the circle of Willis sufficiently to allow detection of intracranial aneurysms as small as 3 to 4 mm.[13] Another study agreed that CTA and MRA have yielded a detection rate of aneurysms measuring at least 4 mm in diameter approaching the detection rate of DSA.[20] The authors cautioned that to avoid diagnostic mishaps, these imaging studies should be reviewed by at least 1 neuroradiologist before aneurysm is rejected as the cause of the oculomotor palsy or before the patient undergoes DSA.[20] Therefore, these imaging studies have, at their best, the capability to detect aneurysms as small as 4 mm, but what is the average size of an aneurysm causing a compressive isolated third nerve palsy. In a retrospective review of 417 cases with posterior communicating artery aneurysmal third nerve palsy, patients were classified based on the results of the noninvasive neuroimaging obtained at initial presentation. The average size of posterior communicating artery aneurysms causing an isolated third nerve palsy was 7.3 mm. This study, also concluded that, aside from an accurate history, the training and experience of the interpreting radiologist is probably the most important factor in determining the reliability of a noninvasive scan in patients with isolated third nerve palsies.[12]

Another group of investigators evaluated the sensitivity and specificity of MRA in the diagnosis of ruptured and unruptured intracranial aneurysms using a metaanalysis. They found 12 studies from 4 electronic databases on relevant articles published from January 1998 to October 2013. Among the 960 patients assessed, a TOF MRA technique was used in most of the studies and showed comparable diagnostic performance to contrast-enhanced MRA. Among studies using 3-T field strength, both sensitivity and specificity were higher compared with studies using lower field strength. They also concluded that MRA is comparable with CTA in diagnosing intracranial aneurysms yet the specificity of MRA seems to be slightly lower than the specificity of CTA.[31] CTA may not detect a thrombosed aneurysm that an MRA will detect (**Fig. 12**). In addition, slow flow components of giant aneurysms or partially

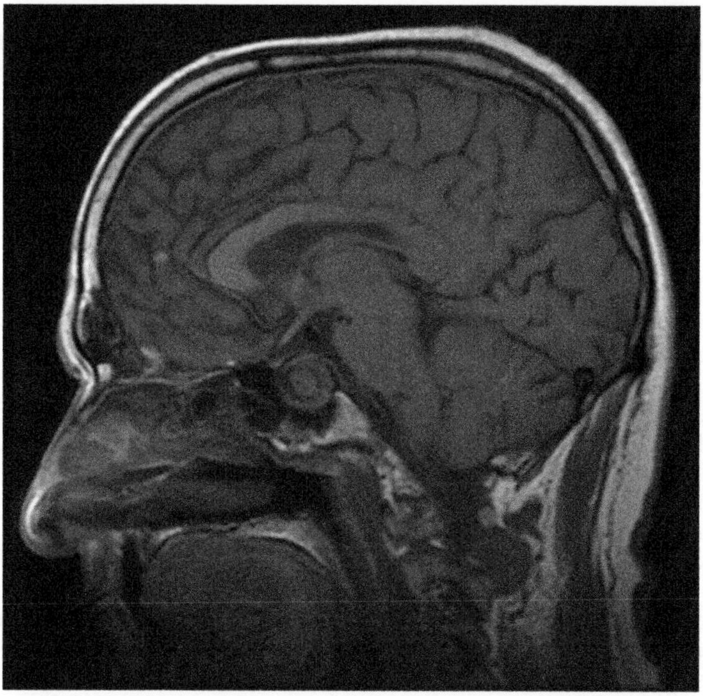

Fig. 12. Sagittal T1 unenhanced scan showing the partially thrombosed aneurysm in the sellar area.

thrombosed aneurysms may also be missed with MRA[32] but detected with steady-state MRI (a technique found to be superior to MRA for delineating and characterizing intraluminal thrombus within aneurysms).[33] If there is a question of a cause of the third cranial palsy other than an intracranial aneurysm, like a third cranial nerve schwannoma, orbital pseudotumor or ophthalmoplegic migraine, than contrast-enhanced MRI is superior in showing enhancing pathology over CTA and obviously DSA. Also, MRA has an important role in the follow-up of aneurysms after endovascular embolization because of its high reliability in the display residual flow within the coil mesh or in the neck region of the aneurysm.[32]

SUMMARY

In a patient with an oculomotor palsy, CTA is generally more sensitive than MRA in the detection of aneurysms. At their best, both modalities have the capability to detect aneurysms as small as 4 mm in diameter. DSA can detect aneurysms smaller than 3 mm in diameter, yet most reports have maintained that a posterior communicating artery aneurysm needs to be at least 4 mm to cause a third nerve palsy. For best results, these imaging studies should be reviewed by at least 1 neuroradiologist. If an aneurysm is not the only pathology in the differential diagnosis of the third cranial nerve palsy, then the combination of MRA and CTA is more powerful than either technique alone. Unfortunately, for logistical and insurance purposes, it is usually easier and more economical to obtain an MRI and MRA than an MRI and CTA because MRI and CTA require 2 separate machines. The other option is to obtain the CTA and inspect the maximum intensity projection images for structural lesions along the course of the oculomotor cranial nerve. However, this technique may not display subtle oculomotor cranial nerve or cavernous sinus enhancement seen in some inflammatory disorders, which MRI would detect. Finally, DSA is still the definitive modality when evaluating for intracranial aneurysms; however, many institutions are using only CTA in the diagnosis and treatment of intracranial aneurysms.

REFERENCES

1. Vaphiades MS, Horton JA. MRA or CTA, that's the question. Surv Ophthalmol 2005;50:406–10.
2. Kissel JT, Burde RM, Klingele TG, et al. Pupil-sparing oculomotor palsies with internal carotid-posterior communicating artery aneurysms. Ann Neurol 1983;13:149–54.
3. Trobe JD. Third nerve palsy and the pupil. Footnotes to the rule. Arch Ophthalmol 1988;106:601–2.
4. Trobe JD. Managing oculomotor nerve palsy. Arch Ophthalmol 1998;116:798.
5. Jacobson DM. Pupil involvement in patients with diabetes-associated oculomotor nerve palsy. Arch Ophthalmol 1998;116:723–7.
6. Jacobson DM. Relative pupil-sparing third nerve palsy: etiology and clinical variables predictive of a mass. Neurology 2001;56:797–8.
7. Yousem DM, Grossman RI. Neuroradiology: the requisites. 3rd edition. Philadelphia: Mosby, Inc; 2010. p. 13, 160–3.
8. Mayberg MR, Batjer HH, Dacey R, et al. Guidelines for the management of aneurysmal subarachnoid hemorrhage. A statement for healthcare professionals from a special writing group of the stroke council, American heart association. Circulation 1994;90:2592–605.
9. Orz Y, AlYamany M. The impact of size and location on rupture of intracranial aneurysms. Asian J Neurosurg 2015;10:26–31.
10. The international study of unruptured intracranial aneurysms investigators. Unruptured intracranial aneurysms–risk of rupture and risks of surgical intervention. N Engl J Med 1998;339:1725–33.
11. Wiebers DO, Whisnant JP, Huston J 3rd, et al. Unruptured intracranial aneurysms: natural history, clinical outcome, and risks of surgical and endovascular treatment. Lancet 2003;362:103–10.
12. Elmalem VI, Hudgins PA, Bruce BB, et al. Underdiagnosis of posterior communicating artery aneurysm in noninvasive brain vascular studies. J Neuroophthalmol 2011;31:103–9.
13. Ross JS, Masaryk TJ, Modic MT, et al. Intracranial aneurysms: evaluation by MR Angiography. AJNR Am J Neuroradiol 1990;11:449–56.
14. White PM, Wardlaw JM. Unruptured intracranial aneurysms. J Neuroradiol 2003; 30:336–50.
15. Jacobson DM, Trobe JD. The emerging role of magnetic resonance angiography in the management of patients with third cranial nerve palsy. Am J Ophthalmol 1999;28:94–6.
16. Lee AG, Hayman LA, Brazis PW. The evaluation of isolated third nerve palsy revisited: an update on the evolving role of magnetic resonance, computed tomography, and catheter angiography. Surv Ophthalmol 2002;47:137–57.
17. Anderson GB, Ashforth R, Steinke DE, et al. CT angiography for the detection and characterization of carotid artery bifurcation disease. Stroke 2000;31:2168–74.
18. Thiex R, Norbash AM, Frerichs KU. The safety of dedicated-team catheter-based diagnostic cerebral angiography in the era of advanced noninvasive imaging. AJNR Am J Neuroradiol 2010;31:230–4.

19. Villablanca JP, Jahan R, Hooshi P, et al. Detection and characterization of very small cerebral aneurysms by using 2D and 3D helical CT angiography. AJNR Am J Neuroradiol 2002;23:1187–98.
20. Chaudhary N, Davagnanam I, Ansari SA, et al. Imaging of intracranial aneurysms causing isolated third cranial nerve palsy. J Neuroophthalmol 2009;29:238–44.
21. El Khaldi M, Pernter P, Ferro F, et al. Detection of cerebral aneurysms in nontraumatic subarachnoid haemorrhage: role of multislice CT angiography in 130 consecutive patients. Radiol Med 2007;112:123–37.
22. Menke J, Larsen J, Kallenberg K. Diagnosing cerebral aneurysms by computed tomographic angiography: meta-analysis. Ann Neurol 2011;69:646–54.
23. Tang K, Li R, Lin J, et al. The value of cerebral CT angiography with low tube voltage in detection of intracranial aneurysms. Biomed Res Int 2015;2015: 876796.
24. Ringelstein A, Lechel U, Fahrendorf DM, et al. Radiation exposure in perfusion CT of the brain. J Comput Assist Tomogr 2014;38:25–8.
25. Brenner D, Elliston C, Hall E, et al. Estimated risks of radiation-induced fatal cancer from pediatric CT. AJR Am J Roentgenol 2001;176:289–96.
26. Prokop M, Debatin JF. MRI contrast media: new developments and trends. CTA vs. MRA. Eur Radiol 1997;7(Suppl 5):299–306.
27. Kaufman DI. Magnetic resonance angiography, computed tomographic angiography, conventional angiography: when to use and why. Recent advances in brain angiography and the impact on neuro-ophthalmology. AAO Neuro-Ophthalmology Subspecialty Day Course Syllabus; 2001. p. 47–52.
28. Jäger HR, Grieve JP. Advances in non-invasive imaging of intracranial vascular disease. Ann R Coll Surg Engl 2000;82:1–5.
29. Balcer LJ, Galetta SL, Yousem DM, et al. Pupil-involving third nerve palsy and carotid stenosis: rapid recovery following endarterectomy. Ann Neurol 1997;41: 273–6.
30. Kupersmith MJ, Heller G, Cox TA. Magnetic resonance angiography and clinical evaluation of third nerve palsies and posterior communicating artery aneurysms. J Neurosurg 2006;105:228–34.
31. Sailer AM, Wagemans BA, Nelemans PJ, et al. Diagnosing intracranial aneurysms with MR angiography: systematic review and meta-analysis. Stroke 2014;45: 119–26.
32. Stafa A, Leonardi M. Role of neuroradiology in evaluating cerebral aneurysms. Interv Neuroradiol 2008;14(Suppl 1):23–37.
33. Martin AJ, Hetts SW, Dillon WP, et al. Imaging of partially thrombosed cerebral aneurysms: characteristics and evolution. AJNR Am J Neuroradiol 2011;32: 346–51.

Update on Ocular Myasthenia Gravis

Stacy V. Smith, MD[a], Andrew G. Lee, MD[a,b,c,d,e,f,g,h,*]

KEYWORDS

• Myasthenia gravis • Diplopia • Ptosis • Ophthalmoplegia • Weakness
• Autoimmune disease • Neuromuscular junction disorder

KEY POINTS

- The clinical presentation of ocular myasthenia gravis (OMG) includes any pattern or combination of pupil sparing ophthalmoplegia, with or without ptosis.
- The differential diagnosis of OMG includes other neurogenic (supranuclear, internuclear, ocular motor cranial neuropathy) or myogenic (orbital restrictive or mechanical disease) etiologies of ptosis and/or ophthalmoplegia.
- The recommended diagnostic modalities for patients suspected of having OMG clinically include serologic testing, chest imaging for thymoma, and electrophysiologic testing and/or single fiber electromyography.
- Although there is no cure for OMG, recommended treatments include acetylcholinesterase inhibitors (eg, pyridostigmine), immunosuppression (eg, prednisone), and thymectomy (especially if a thymoma is present).
- The prognosis for OMG is variable; acute/subacute symptomatic and conservative treatment is useful, but some patients require more aggressive and longer term immunosuppression.

Disclosures: None of the authors have any relevant disclosures.
[a] Department of Ophthalmology, Blanton Eye Institute, Houston Methodist Hospital, Scurlock Tower, 6560 Fannin Street, Suite 450, Houston, TX 77030, USA; [b] Baylor College of Medicine, 1 Baylor Plaza, Houston, TX 77030, USA; [c] Department of Ophthalmology, University of Texas Medical Branch (UTMB), Galveston, TX, USA; [d] Department of Ophthalmology, Weill Cornell Medicine, New York, NY, USA; [e] Department of Neurology, Weill Cornell Medicine, New York, NY, USA; [f] Department of Neurosurgery, Weill Cornell Medicine, New York, NY, USA; [g] Section of Ophthalmology, UT MD Anderson Cancer Center (UTMDACC), Houston, TX, USA; [h] Department of Ophthalmology, University of Iowa Hospitals and Clinics, Iowa City, IA, USA
* Corresponding author. Department of Ophthalmology, Blanton Eye Institute, Houston Methodist Hospital, Scurlock Tower, 6560 Fannin Street, Suite 450, Houston, TX 77030.
E-mail address: AGLee@HoustonMethodist.org

Neurol Clin 35 (2017) 115–123
http://dx.doi.org/10.1016/j.ncl.2016.08.008

INTRODUCTION

Ocular myasthenia gravis (OMG) is a localized form of the autoimmune disorder myasthenia gravis (MG) in which antibodies directed against acetylcholine receptors (AChR) block or destroy these receptors at the postsynaptic neuromuscular junction (eg, binding, blocking, modulating AChR antibodies). Many patients with OMG, however, have no detectable AChR antibodies (ie, seronegative MG). Commonly, OMG produces ocular symptoms of painless ptosis and/or diplopia by affecting one or more extraocular muscles. For all forms of MG the incidence is 0.04 to 5 per 100,000 per year and the estimated prevalence is 0.5 to 12.5 per 100,000 per year.[1] MG affects all age groups, genders, and ethnicities; however, OMG shows a predilection for men.[1] In this article, we review the most recent literature concerning the clinical presentation, differential diagnosis, diagnostic modalities, treatment, and prognosis of OMG.

CLINICAL PRESENTATION

The hallmark of OMG is a history of weakness or fatigability of the extraocular muscles and/or ptosis with normal pupillary function, sensory function, and visual acuity. The weakness is often variable and increases with repeated or sustained muscle use throughout the day (ie, fatigability) and improves with rest, sleep, and cold temperature.[2,3] As outlined in **Table 1**, weakness of specific muscles can mimic other supranuclear, internuclear, or infranuclear efferent system abnormalities and can be unilateral or bilateral.[2,4] Evoli and colleagues[5] found that ptosis and levator palpebrae superioris weakness was the only presenting sign in roughly 10% of patients in their study of OMG. Ptosis of 1 lid may be enhanced by passively elevating the contralateral lid (ie, enhancement of ptosis) and is due to the bilateral and equal innervation (Hering's law of equal innervation) of the lids.[6] Ptosis and extraocular muscle weakness may become more pronounced (ie, fatigable ptosis) if the patient sustains upward gaze for a prolonged period.[4]

Another characteristic sign of OMG is the Cogan's lid twitch sign, in which the lid briefly elevates excessively after a vertical saccade from a downgaze position. The Cogan's lid twitch can also occur spontaneously. Occasionally, more persistent eye lid retraction can also be seen with OMG. This "pseudoretraction" in OMG is due to excessive stimulation of the normal lid attempting to compensate for the drooping of the lid of the opposite eye (again, owing to the bilateral equal innervation of Hering's law).[4] Pseudoretraction can be differentiated from true retraction in this setting by having the examiner manually elevate the ptotic eye lid to determine if there is resolution (pseudoretraction) or lack of resolution (true lid retraction) of the retracted eyelid.[4] Pseudoretraction and true lid retraction, however, are not specific for OMG and may be present in other disorders like Lambert-Eaton myasthenic syndrome, thyroid eye disease, age related levator dehiscence associated ptosis, ocular myopathy, Fisher syndrome, and third nerve palsy.[7–9]

Table 1
Muscles impaired in ocular myasthenia gravis

Muscle	Finding
Levator palpebrae superioris	Unilateral or bilateral ptosis
Extraocular muscles	Any pattern of unilateral or bilateral, painless, pupil-spared ophthalmoplegia
Orbicularis oculi	"Peek" sign; ectropion, orbicularis weakness

OMG may selectively impair any single or combination of extraocular muscle(s), but very commonly affects the medial rectus.[2] This leads to similarities in presentation between OMG and many other motor cranial nerve palsies that spare the pupil.[2,4,10] Pseudointranuclear ophthalmoplegia, pseudo-one-and-a-half syndrome, complete external ophthalmoplegia, divergence and convergence pareses, and double elevator palsy have all been described in MG.[2,4,9,11,12] Abnormalities in saccadic eye movements may also be observed in OMG, including hypermetric saccades, intersaccadic fatigue leading to undershoot of target, jerky or quivering eye movements, and gaze-evoked nystagmus.[2,4,9] Thus, OMG should be considered in the differential diagnosis of any pattern of painless, unilateral or bilateral, pupil-sparing ophthalmoplegia with or without ptosis.

Clinicians should also test orbicularis muscle function in patients with suspected OMG. Bilateral orbicularis weakness is commonly seen in patients with OMG and would not be expected in other non–MG-related etiologies of diplopia/ophthalmoplegia (eg, ocular motor cranial neuropathy or thyroid eye disease). During sustained forceful eye closure, patients with orbicularis oculi involvement may develop a "peek sign" with orbicularis oculi fatigue leading to partial opening of palpebral fissure.[2,4] Lower eyelid ectropion can also occur, especially with repetitive use and strain throughout the day.[4,9]

DIFFERENTIAL DIAGNOSIS

The differential diagnosis of OMG is outlined in **Box 1**. In addition, the diagnosis of generalized MG (GMG) should also be considered in all patients presenting with OMG. Systemic symptoms include difficulty swallowing, difficulty chewing food, change in voice, shortness of breath, and weakness in the extremities. The management of OMG is often best achieved with a multidisciplinary approach and we recommend that eye doctors consider referring their patients with OMG for comanagement, GMG evaluation, and systemic treatment with a neurologist. Likewise, neurologists might consider the assistance of an ophthalmologist for evaluating, monitoring, and treating symptomatically or surgically any ptosis and diplopia symptoms that do not respond to maximum medical therapy for the MG.

DIAGNOSTIC MODALITIES

MG is a clinical diagnosis supported by ancillary laboratory, imaging, and electrophysiologic testing. Although there are several diagnostic tests available for the evaluation of MG, there is no single test that can establish an absolute diagnosis of MG and there

Box 1
Differential diagnosis of myasthenia gravis

Thyroid eye disease

Chronic progressive external ophthalmoplegia

Mitochondrial myopathy (Kearns-Sayre disease)

Muscular dystrophy

Levator dehiscence

Single and multiple cranial nerve neuropathy (III, IV, VI)

Data from Refs.[2,4,7–10]

is no test to "rule out" MG. Diagnostic tests are used to help support a clinical diagnosis made on the history and physical examination, and can be categorized as clinical, laboratory (serologic), electrophysiologic, and pharmacologic.[9,13]

The fatigue test, sleep test, and ice test are the 3 currently available clinical tests for MG (**Table 2**). One bedside clinical test is the fatigue test and although highly suggestive of MG, it is not 100% specific.[13] The patient is instructed to sustain upward gaze followed by the development of worsening ptosis or diplopia from eyelid and extraocular muscle fatigue.[13] The sleep and rest tests are based on the principle that the symptoms of MG worsen with fatigue and improve after a period of rest.[14] According to Odel and colleagues, patients demonstrated an immediate resolution of ptosis and ophthalmoplegia after a 30-minute period of quiet sleep, followed by the reappearance of MG signs over the next 30 seconds to 5 minutes. The test is relatively specific but only moderately sensitive.[14] The ice test is another easy, safe, and effective clinical test that works on the principle of muscle strengthening upon local cooling. By simply placing an icepack over the eyelids for several minutes, patients with MG may show a transient improvement in ptosis.[13] The tests are not mutually exclusive and some authors believe that the ice test is an enhanced rest test. Although very specific, the ice test is only relatively sensitive, because some MG patients with ptosis (especially complete ptosis) may fail to respond.[13] Serologic screening for circulating autoantibodies to the nicotinic AChRs (anti-AChR antibodies) can be positive in up to 80% to 90% of patients with GMG.[13] However, AChR antibody testing only has a sensitivity of 50% to 60% in OMG as compared with GMG.[13] Evoli and colleagues[5] reports a study on 48 patients with pure OMG, of which only 45.5% had detectable anti-AChR antibodies. Additional autoantibodies such as the anti–muscle-specific kinase antibody may be positive in seronegative cases.[15]

Table 2
Tests for myasthenia gravis

Test Name	Positive Result	Statistics
Sleep or rest test	Improving symptoms after a period of rest	Moderate sensitivity and specificity
Ice test	Improvement of ptosis after icepack is applied to the eyelids for several minutes	Moderately sensitive and high specificity
Fatigue test	Eyelid fatigue with upward gaze	High specificity
Serologic test for anti-AChR antibodies	Positive for anti-AChR antibodies (binding, blocking, and modulating forms)	Moderate sensitivity but high specificity
Repetitive nerve stimulation	Decrement in compound muscle action potential of stimulated nerves	Low sensitivity and high specificity
Single fiber EMG	Abnormal jitter of weak muscles	High sensitivity but may not be universally available
Edrophonium test	Symptom improvement with edrophonium	High sensitivity and specificity but largely supplanted by less invasive clinical and laboratory tests discussed

Abbreviations: AChR, acetylcholine receptors; EMG, electromyography.
Data from Refs.[15,16,18,19]

In addition to serologic testing, electromyography (EMG) can be used to support a clinical diagnosis of MG especially in seronegative MG. Repetitive nerve stimulation can be performed as part of the EMG study. Proximal and facial nerves are repetitively stimulated, and fluctuations in the amplitude and duration of the motor unit potentials are recorded. Patients with MG are expected to show a decrement in the compound muscle action potential of the stimulated nerves.[16] Repetitive nerve stimulation has low sensitivity (18%–35%) in OMG, but relatively high specificity.[13] Some potential errors can occur during testing owing to poor technique or minimal involvement of the muscle being tested.[13] The frequency of stimulation can vary, and lower frequency stimulation of 2 to 3 Hz is commonly used to detect MG. In contrast with typical MG, when assessing for Lambert-Eaton myasthenic syndrome, the technician must use a much higher frequency of stimulation and patients with Lambert-Eaton myasthenic syndrome often show incremental rather than decremental EMG responses.

Single fiber EMG is more sensitive (80%–88%) than traditional EMG or repetitive nerve stimulation. Up to 99% of MG patients show an abnormal jitter will be noted on single fiber EMG.[17] Although the extensor digitorum communis is found to be abnormal in most patients with MG, the muscles tested should be based on the patient's distribution of weakness.[17] False-positive results may arise owing to other neuromuscular disorders or owing to poor technique.[13] The single fiber EMG remains the gold standard electrophysiologic test for diagnosis of MG, but requires specialized skill and is not readily available in many care centers. It is especially useful in seronegative MG cases where a definitive diagnosis is needed to proceed with therapy.

Edrophonium chloride (Enlon, Mylan Institutional, Rockford, IL, USA; Tensilon, formerly manufactured by Valeant Pharmaceuticals, Laval, Quebec, Canada) is a short-acting reversible acetylcholinesterase inhibitor that can be used in the evaluation of suspected MG. Intravenous edrophonium transiently increases the availability of acetylcholine at the receptor sites.[13] Intramuscular neostigmine (Prostigmin, Valeant, Laval, Quebec, Canada) was also used in the past for clinical testing of MG and has a longer half-life for measuring diplopia/ophthalmoplegia orthoptic endpoints. It is 86% sensitive in OMG patients and 95% sensitive in GMG patients.[13] However, the edrophonium test has a potential for adverse cardiovascular effects and should be used with caution in patients with heart disease or in patients on atrioventricular node–blocking drugs such as digoxin or beta blockers.[13] The test can also be complicated by cholinergic side effects. Therefore, the edrophonium and neostigmine tests have been increasingly supplanted by the noninvasive rest/sleep and/or ice tests.[13]

Although MG should be suspected in patients with any pattern of neurologically isolated, unilateral or bilateral, pupil-sparing, ophthalmoparesis, neuroimaging studies (eg, computed tomography and MRI) should be performed to rule out intracranial lesions in atypical cases (eg, strictly unilateral and seronegative). Patients with clinical OMG with positive AChR antibody, eletrophysiologic, ice/rest/sleep, or edrophonium testing may not require neuroimaging.[4] Additionally, computed tomography or MRI of the mediastinum should be performed in OMG patients even though the risk of thymoma is only 4% in OMG patients, compared with a 12% risk in patients with GMG.[9,18]

TREATMENT OPTIONS FOR OCULAR MYASTHENIA GRAVIS

Treatment of OMG depends on the severity of the symptoms at time of presentation. Many mild OMG symptoms (eg, ptosis or intermittent diplopia) can be managed with nonmedical treatments such as patching, lid crutch attachment to the spectacle frame, and taping of the affected eyelid.[19] Medical therapy for ptosis should be pursued if the patient does not have resolution or marked improvement of symptoms with nonmedical treatment.[19,20] Surgical ptosis repair can be considered if patients are symptomatic, stable, and have failed conservative and medical treatments.

Cholinesterase inhibitors such as pyridostigmine (Mestinon, Valeant) remain the first-line treatment for symptomatic relief.[19,20] Ptosis may improve the most with cholinesterase usage; however, symptoms of diplopia may have little to no response.[21] Benator and colleagues[22] report a randomized trial of patients with OMG who were treated concurrently with pyridostigmine and prednisone. Data from the study showed that pyridostigmine alone failed to cause remission of the disease.[22]

In addition to pyridostigmine, another potential treatment for OMG is corticosteroid therapy. Low and moderate dose corticosteroids have been shown to improve diplopia in OMG and there has been some anecdotal evidence to support the use of steroids to reduce the frequency of deterioration to GMG. The long-term side effects of corticosteroids may limit their use for chronic MG.[21,23] Epidemiologic historical studies have demonstrated that the progression of OMG to GMG was 60% before the use of immunosuppressants, compared with 30% after the introduction of immunosuppressant therapy.[24] Kupersmith and colleagues[21] were among the first to advocate that low-dose corticosteroids or other forms of immunosuppressive therapy (eg, azathioprine, mycophenolate mofetil, methotrexate) may also play a role in preventing disease progression in OMG.[23] They reported a retrospective study of 32 patients with OMG who were treated with prednisone and followed for a minimum of 2 years. Patients were treated with a high initial dose of 40 to 80 mg prednisone, which was tapered over a course of 4 to 6 weeks. This was followed by a 2.5- to 20-mg dose of prednisone given on alternate days. At 2 years, diplopia was found to be absent in 21 of the 29 patients who initially had this finding. Furthermore, the frequency of deterioration to GMG was 9.4% and only occurred in 3 patients. None of the patients were reported to have any complications from use of corticosteroids.[21,23] The EPITOME (Efficacy of Prednisone for the Treatment of Ocular Myasthenia) trial was a randomized controlled trial set to assess the safety and determine the risks and benefits of low- and high-dose steroid therapy to prevent progression of OMG to GMG. This trial was able to demonstrate the safety of low dose-steroid therapy, but could not generate sufficient evidence for the use of high-dose steroid therapy in delaying disease progression owing to low participant accrual.[22] Current recommendations advocate the use of cholinesterase inhibitors, followed by low-dose steroid use if cholinesterase treatment alone does not control symptoms adequately.[21,25]

Steroid-sparing agents such as azathioprine, methotrexate, and mycophenolate mofetil may be added to the regimen if steroid treatment does not alleviate symptoms.[21,26] Cyclophosphamide, cyclosporine, intravenous immunoglobulin, and plasmapheresis can be considered but usually are not required for OMG.[20]

Thymectomy in MG is indicated in the presence of thymoma, but there remains debate as to whether or not it should be used in OMG when no thymoma is present.[27] Thymectomy without thymoma has had some success in the treatment of GMG, but there is still reluctance to pursue thymectomy for pure OMG.[27] Nakamura and colleagues[28] demonstrated that thymectomy in OMG was most effective if patients underwent surgery within 12 months of symptoms. A recent trial published in 2011 by Liu and colleagues[29] retrospectively reviewed 115 patients who were treated with thymectomy for OMG after they were either unresponsive to pyridostigmine treatment, found to have a thymoma, or had relapsed after immunosuppressive therapy. In this study, 26.4% of patients were asymptomatic after 12 months, not requiring any medical intervention, and 58.2% showed improvement in symptoms.[29] The authors, however, acknowledged that a clinical trial comparing medical therapy with surgery is still needed to definitively determine if thymectomy is an appropriate early intervention.

Nevertheless, it is reasonable to consider thymectomy in the absence of thymoma after failing other medical therapies in MG. The risks of the operative procedure itself and the use anesthetic agents in a patient with neuromuscular disease must be discussed with the patient.

PROGNOSIS OF OCULAR MYASTHENIA GRAVIS

The prognosis of OMG is generally good with the combination use of short-term corticosteroids with or without pyridostigmine. As noted, longer term steroid-sparing regimens (eg, azathioprine) have also been useful in OMG. Sommer and colleagues[30] reported remission in most of their treated patients with OMG and the frequency of patients developing GMG was decreased with the use of this combination therapy. MG was confined to the extraocular muscles in 69% of patients, of which 54% were in remission, 33% improved, and 13% remained unchanged. Furthermore, 31% of patients progressed to GMG, which is a relatively low fraction compared with the 49% to 69% reported in previous studies.

For patients with diplopia resistant to medical therapy, prism or occlusion therapy is an option.[19,20] If the ocular deviation is large or not satisfactorily treated with conservative measures, then strabismus surgery may be recommended once ocular misalignment measurements have been stable for 6 months.[4] The prognosis after strabismus surgery in OMG is variable, but some reports have shown up to 50% remission rates and others report a worse long-term prognosis.[31–33] Similarly, persistent ptosis in MG can be surgically repaired, but the outcomes are variable. The potential benefits of surgery must be weighed against the increased risk for recurrence after surgery and the potential for worsening MG or respiratory failure with anesthetic agents.

SUMMARY

OMG should be considered in patients with any pattern of unilateral or bilateral, pupil-spared, painless, diplopia, ptosis, or ophthalmoplegia. We recommend neuroimaging for atypical cases (eg, strictly unilateral OMG). Serologic, radiographic, and electrophysiologic testing support the clinical diagnosis of OMG. Although cholinesterase inhibitors can provide symptomatic relief, disease modification with corticosteroids or longer term immunosuppression (eg, azathioprine) may be better for symptom control in OMG and may reduce conversion of OMG to GMG. Strabismus and ptosis surgery may be considered in patients who fail medical and conservative therapy and have stable measurements.

ACKNOWLEDGMENTS

Ernest R. Pucketta, Saagar N. Patela, Karima Khimania are acknowledged for their significant role in literature review and manuscript composition for this article.

REFERENCES

1. Vaphiades MS, Bhatti MT, Lesser RL. Ocular myasthenia gravis. Curr Opin Ophthalmol 2012;23:537–42.
2. Weinberg DA, Lesser RL, Vollmer TL. Ocular myasthenia: a protean disorder. Surv Ophthalmol 1994;39:169–210.
3. Golnik KC, Pena R, Lee AG, et al. An ice test for the diagnosis of myasthenia gravis. Ophthalmology 1999;106:1282.
4. Miller NR. Walsh and Hoyt's clinical neuro-ophthalmology. 4th edition. Baltimore (MD): Williams & Wilkins; 1985. p. 841–91.

5. Evoli A, Tonali P, Bartoccioni AP, et al. Ocular myasthenia: diagnostic and therapeutic problems. Acta Neurol Scand 1988;77:31–5.
6. Averbuch-Heller L, Poonyathalang A, von Maydell RD, et al. Hering's law for eyelids: still valid. Neurology 1995;45:1781–3.
7. Bravis PW. Enhanced ptosis in Lambert-Eaton myasthenic syndrome. J Neuroophthalmol 1997;17:202–3.
8. Ishikawa H, Wakakura M, Ishikawa S. Enhanced ptosis in Fisher's syndrome after Epstein-Barr virus infection. J Clin Neuroophthalmol 1990;10:197–200.
9. Lee AG, Brazis PW. Ocular myasthenia gravis. In: Lee AG, Brazis PW, editors. Clinical pathways in neuro-ophthalmology: an evidence based approach. 2nd edition. New York: Thieme; 2003. p. 337–48.
10. Dehaene I, van Zandijcke M. Isolated paralysis of the superior division of the ocular motor nerve mimicked by myasthenic gravis. Neuroophthalmololgy 1995;15:257–8.
11. Bandini F, Faga D, Simonetti S. Ocular myasthenia mimicking a one-and-a-half syndrome. J Neuroophthalmol 2001;21:210–1.
12. Lepore FE. Divergence paresis: a nonlocalizing cause of diplopia. J Neuroophthalmol 1999;19:242–5.
13. Okun MS, Charriez CM, Bhatti MT, et al. Tensilon and the diagnosis of myasthenia gravis: are we using the tensilon test too much? Neurologist 2001;7:295–9.
14. Odel J, Winterkorn J, Behrens M. The sleep test for myasthenia gravis—a safe alternative to Tensilon. J Clin Neuro-ophthalmol 1991;11:288–92.
15. Bennett DLH, Mills KR, Riordan-Eva P, et al. Anti-MuSK antibodies in a case of ocular myasthenia gravis. J Neurol Neurosurg Psychiatry 2006;77:564–5.
16. Hermann RC Jr. Repetitive stimulation studies. In: Daube JR, editor. Clinical neurophysiology. Philadelphia: FA Davis; 1996. p. 237–47.
17. Sanders DB, Howard JF. Single fiber EMG in myasthenia gravis. Muscle Nerve 1986;9:809–19.
18. Papetestas AE, Genkins G, Horowitz SH, et al. Studies in myasthenia gravis: effects of thymectomy. Results in 1985 patients with nonthymomatous and thymomatous myasthenia gravis, 1941-1969. Am J Med 1971;50:465–76.
19. Haines SR, Thurtell MJ. Treatment of ocular myasthenia gravis. Curr Treat Options Neurol 2012;14:103–12.
20. Kerty E, Elsais A, Argov Z, et al. EFNS/ENS guidelines for treatment of ocular myasthenia. Eur J Neurol 2014;21:687–93.
21. Kupersmith MJ, Moster M, Bhuiyan S, et al. Beneficial effects of corticosteroids on ocular myasthenia gravis. Arch Neurol 1996;53:802–4.
22. Benator M, McDermott MP, Sanders DB, et al. Efficacy of Prednisone for the treatment of Ocular Myasthenia (EPITOME): a randomized, controlled trial. Muscle Nerve 2016;53:363–9.
23. Kupersmith MJ. Ocular myasthenia gravis treatment: treatment success and failures in patients with long-term follow up. J Neurol 2009;256:1314–20.
24. Wong SH, Plant GT, Cornblath W. Does treatment of ocular myasthenia gravis with early immunosuppressive therapy prevent secondarily generalization and should it be offered to all such patients? J Neuroophthalmol 2016;36:98–102.
25. Kaminski HJ, Daroff RB. Treatment of ocular myasthenia. Steroids only when compelled. Arch Neurol 2000;57:752–3.
26. Mee J, Paine M, Byrne E, et al. Immunotherapy of ocular myasthenia gravis reduces conversion to generalized myasthenia gravis. J Neuroophthalmol 2003;23:251–5.

27. Lanska DJ. Indications for thymectomy in myasthenia gravis. Neurology 1990;40: 1828–9.
28. Nakamura H, Taniguchi Y, Suzuki Y, et al. Delayed remission after thymectomy for myasthenia gravis of the purely ocular type. J Thorac Cardiovasc Surg 1996;112: 371–5.
29. Liu Z, Feng H, Yeung S-CJ, et al. Extended transsternal thymectomy for the treatment of ocular myasthenia gravis. Ann Thorac Surg 2011;92:1993–9.
30. Sommer N, Sigg B, Melms A, et al. Ocular myasthenia gravis: response to long term immunosuppressive treatment. J Neurol Neurosurg Psychiatry 1997;62: 156–62.
31. Morris OC, O'Day J. Strabismus surgery in the management of diplopia caused by myasthenia gravis. Br J Ophthalmol 2004;88:832.
32. Bentley CR, Dawson E, Lee JP. Active management in patients with ocular manifestations of myasthenia gravis. Eye 2001;15:18–22.
33. Bradley E, Bartley G, Chapman K, et al. Surgical correction of blepharoptosis in patients with myasthenia gravis. Ophthal Plast Recons 2001;17:103–10.

Orbital Disease in Neuro-Ophthalmology

Jessica R. Chang, MD, Anna M. Gruener, BMBS, MSc, FRCOphth,
Timothy J. McCulley, MD*

KEYWORDS

- Orbit • Orbital fracture • Traumatic optic neuropathy • Enophthalmos
- Idiopathic orbital inflammatory syndrome • Thyroid eye disease
- IgG4-related disease

KEY POINTS

- Orbital compartment syndrome, cavernous sinus thrombosis, and orbital mucormycosis are neuro-ophthalmologic emergencies.
- Trapdoor fractures may present as acute diplopia without many stigmata of trauma, cannot be diagnosed by CT alone, and require urgent surgery.
- There is no proven effective treatment for traumatic optic neuropathy.
- Enophthalmos may be caused by orbital fracture, silent sinus syndrome, chronic intracranial hypotension, and rare fibrosing diseases.
- Infection must be excluded in cases of orbital inflammation, especially in patients who may be immunocompromised.

INTRODUCTION

Many abnormalities of the orbit present with neuro-ophthalmic findings, such as impaired ocular motility or alignment, and sensory changes, including optic neuropathy. Comprehensive coverage of all orbital diseases is beyond the scope of this article. This review focuses on diagnosis and management of the most common and the most vision- or life-threatening orbital conditions as well as more recently discovered entities and points of active controversy. These conditions include orbital trauma, vascular disease, inflammatory and infectious diseases, and neoplasms. Common presenting symptoms and associated neuro-orbital diseases also are summarized (**Table 1**).

Disclosures: None.
Wilmer Eye Institute, Johns Hopkins University School of Medicine, Baltimore, MD 21287, USA
* Corresponding author. Wilmer Eye Institute, 600 North Wolfe Street, Woods Building #457, Baltimore, MD 21287.
E-mail address: tmccull5@jhmi.edu

Neurol Clin 35 (2017) 125–144
http://dx.doi.org/10.1016/j.ncl.2016.08.011 neurologic.theclinics.com

Table 1
Neuro-ophthalmic manifestations of orbital disease

		Optic Disc Edema and/or Optic Neuropathy
Compressive	Neoplastic	• Primary (eg, optic nerve sheath meningioma, rhabdomyosarcoma) • Secondary (eg, metastasis to extraocular muscle) • Vascular (eg, capillary hemangioma, cavernous hemangioblastoma)
	Inflammatory	• TED (Graves disease, Hashimoto thyroiditis) • Orbital inflammatory disease (eg, sarcoidosis, IgG4-related orbital disease, idiopathic)
Infiltrative	Neoplastic	• Primary (eg, optic nerve glioma) • Secondary (eg, metastatic carcinoma, lymphoma, leukemia)
	Infectious	• Bacterial • Viral • Fungal
	Inflammatory	• Systemic disease (eg, sarcoidosis, SLE, granulomatosis with polyangiitis) • Idiopathic optic perineuritis
Traumatic	Direct	• Impingement or transection from bone fragment or foreign body • Avulsion injury
	Indirect	• Blunt trauma to the forehead or orbit
		Diplopia and/or Motility Abnormality
Mechanical		• Orbital fracture (with or without enophthalmos) • Silent sinus syndrome • Sagging eye, sunken brain syndrome • Globe dystopia from mass lesion (eg, vascular tumor)
Inflammatory		• Myositis • TED • Orbital inflammation (eg, IOIS, IgG4-RD, orbital cellulitis)
Neuropathic		• Infiltrative (inflammatory or neoplastic) • Compressive (eg, cavernous sinus or orbital apex syndrome)
Myopathic		• Chronic progressive external ophthalmoplegia • Congenital fibrosis syndrome

ORBITAL TRAUMA

Orbital fractures are common and may present with periocular swelling, proptosis, enophthalmos, ecchymosis, chemosis, subconjunctival hemorrhage, infraorbital nerve hypoesthesia, diplopia, and decreased vision. One should first assess for globe rupture and orbital compartment syndrome, because emergent intervention for these conditions carries the potential to reverse or prevent permanent vision loss. The treatment of traumatic optic neuropathy (TON) is more controversial. Trapdoor fractures constitute another urgent and sometimes challenging diagnosis; comminuted fractures may also present with acute and/or delayed dysmotility and diplopia.[1–4] Ischemic extraocular muscle entrapment requires urgent surgical intervention to reduce the risk of chronic dysmotility.[4] Enophthalmos often results from orbital trauma, but other mechanisms are also described in later discussion.

ORBITAL COMPARTMENT SYNDROME

The most common cause of orbital compartment syndrome is retrobulbar hemorrhage, whether traumatic or iatrogenic from periocular procedures, such as retrobulbar injection or even blepharoplasty (**Fig. 1**).[5] Spontaneous bleeding into a vascular or lymphatic tumor may also present with acutely elevated orbital pressure (OP).[6–9] Other causes include orbital emphysema and rapid growth of a tumor or inflammatory lesion. Orbital emphysema occurs when a patient with acute orbital fracture blows their nose or sneezes: they may force air into the orbit, and the lacerated soft tissue surrounding the fracture may act as a one-way valve, leading to persistently elevated OP. Hemorrhage in the setting of orbital fracture may or may not cause a tense orbit, depending on whether the hemorrhage is able to drain through the fracture or whether it is loculated. After orbital fracture repair or other orbital surgery, a drain is often placed and vision checks are performed in the immediate postoperative period to evaluate for this complication.

Vision loss in orbital compartment syndrome is due to compressive occlusion of the vasculature supplying the optic nerve or retina. Animal studies have suggested that irreversible damage can occur within 90 to 120 minutes from vascular occlusion in the eye or orbit.[10] Several investigations have evaluated OP and associated visual loss. In patients with thyroid eye disease (TED) with related (compressive) optic neuropathies, OPs have been measured between 17 and 40 mm Hg (mean 28.7 mm Hg).[11] Hargaden and colleagues[12] simulated orbital hemorrhage by inflating balloon catheters within the orbits of 16 nonhuman primates for 3 or more hours. When inflated such that intraocular pressure (IOP) was 50 mm Hg or greater, half of the animals suffered irreparable damage. Hayreh and Jonas[13] demonstrated that with clamping of the central retinal artery, permanent visual loss occurred after 105 minutes. In contrast, however, Katz and colleagues[14] described 2 patients with orbital hemorrhage who regained vision following more than 3 hours of no light perception, and therefore, the visual potential of such patients should not be defined by duration of symptoms alone.

MANAGEMENT OF ORBITAL COMPARTMENT SYNDROME

The management of orbital compartment syndromes consists largely of measuring and urgently treating elevated IOP. Canthotomy with cantholysis is often used as an initial attempt at normalizing OP (**Fig. 2**).[15] Close monitoring of vision, IOP, and afferent pupil response is crucial. Definitive treatment may necessitate orbitotomy with

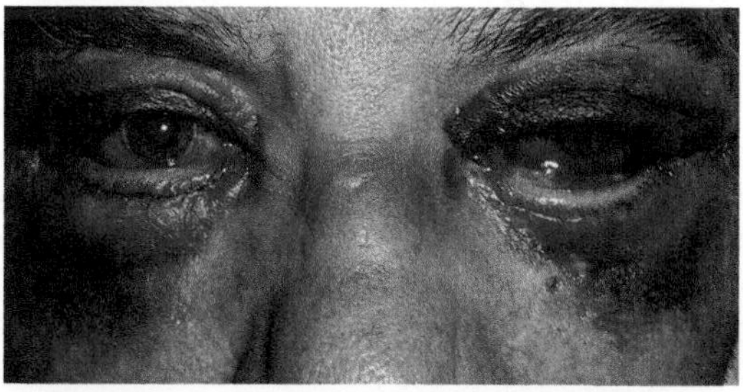

Fig. 1. Orbital hemorrhage after cosmetic blepharoplasty, resulting in loss of vision. (*From* Yoon MK, McCulley TJ. Orbital disease in neuro-ophthalmology. Neurol Clin 2010;28(3): 679–99.)

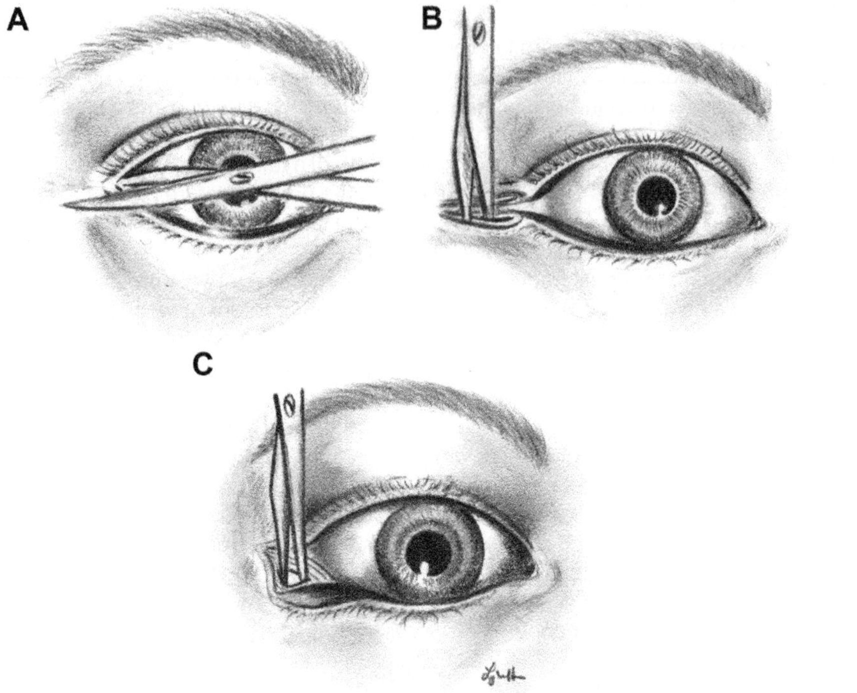

Fig. 2. (A) Canthotomy divides the superior and inferior crura lateral canthal tendon; (*B*) the inferior (and sometimes superior) crux is then lysed; (*C*) blunt dissection achieves septolysis of the orbital septum. (*From* Yoon MK, McCulley TJ. Orbital disease in neuro-ophthalmology. Neurol Clin 2010;28(3):679–99.)

evacuation of a hematoma and control of bleeding through cautery and ligation of vessels; extreme cases may require orbital decompression.

CAROTID-CAVERNOUS SINUS FISTULA

Craniofacial trauma may also result in a direct carotid-cavernous fistula (CCF), most commonly from a basal skull fracture causing a tear in the internal carotid artery within the cavernous sinus.[16] Very rarely, a ruptured intracavernous carotid artery aneurysm may also present acutely with direct CCF. Indirect CCF tends to occur in older patients, with low-flow anastomoses between dural branches of the internal or external carotid artery and the cavernous sinus. Indirect CCF may occur as the result of revascularization after cavernous sinus thrombosis. Patients may present with chemosis, "corkscrew" arterialized episcleral vessels, proptosis (which may be pulsatile), elevated IOP, variable degrees of ophthalmoplegia, and the presence of an orbital bruit (**Fig. 3**). In the absence of trauma, CCF may be mistaken for TED. Cranila and orbital computed tomographic (CT) findings include superior orbital vein engorgement, enlarged extraocular muscles, and sometimes subarachnoid hemorrhage and an enlarged cavernous sinus. CT is preferred in the acute setting, but MRI and magnetic resonance angiography can provide further detail about arterialized blood flow in addition to soft tissue detail; Doppler ultrasound can also provide helpful information

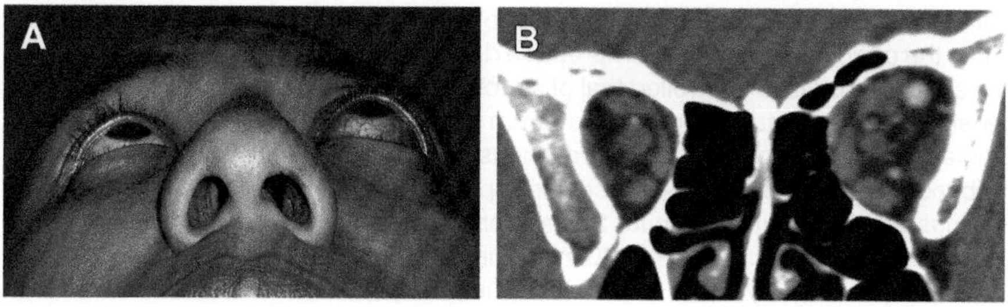

Fig. 3. Carotid cavernous fistula, clinically showing conjunctival injection and proptosis (*A*) and CT shows dilated superior vein and enlarged extraocular muscles (*B*).

about rate and direction of flow, but standard catheter arteriography is the gold standard for defining the critical anatomy of the CCF. Symptomatic direct CCF almost always requires urgent treatment by neurosurgery or interventional radiology.

Cavernous sinus thrombosis is another potential cause of orbital congestion, proptosis, and ophthalmoplegia and constitutes a neuro-ophthalmologic emergency.[17] Sixth nerve paresis is a frequent early sign, but presentation may include corneal anesthesia, Horner syndrome, and even venous stasis retinopathy. Often there is an infectious source, and the patient is acutely ill. Aseptic thrombosis is also possible and usually presents with less severe symptoms.

TRAUMATIC OPTIC NEUROPATHY

Optic neuropathy (in the absence of orbital compartment syndrome) occurs in 0.5% to 5% of orbital traumas.[18] Direct TON occurs when there is disruption of the anatomic integrity of the optic nerve, whether from a foreign body or displaced bone. These injuries are usually associated with severe visual loss and limited therapeutic options. CT scans with fine coronal slices through the optic canal should be obtained on initial evaluation.

Indirect TON is a more common and less obvious diagnosis in which forces are transmitted to the optic nerve from a distance and do not grossly disrupt the anatomy.[19] The most common site of injury is the rigid confined space of the bony optic canal. Some have suggested that force is transmitted through the sphenoid bone causing transient deformation of the canal and contusion of the optic nerve in the canal. Others have suggested that the shock wave from a frontal blow is propagated through the orbital soft tissues and concentrated at the apex by the conical shape of the orbit. Some have suggested initial shearing injury and secondary edema and ischemia in the optic canal, a rigid confined space where the nerve is supplied only by pial vessels.

Indirect TON is diagnosed on clinical examination: visual loss with a relative afferent pupillary defect and otherwise normal globe, including optic nerve appearance (although disc edema may be present). Visual field testing often reveals central or generalized depression, although a variety of optic nerve patterns of visual field loss are possible. Several studies have noted spontaneous improvement after TON in 20% to 50% of cases, with a variable degree of visual acuity recovery.[20,21]

MANAGEMENT OF TRAUMATIC OPTIC NEUROPATHY

Proposed management options include observation, corticosteroids, and optic canal decompression. Several anecdotal studies showed improvement in visual acuity after

TON with corticosteroids.[21,22] The initial rationale was reduction of optic nerve edema within the optic canal, limiting compressive damage to the nerve. There has been only one small randomized controlled trial of steroids for TON, which showed no significant benefit, but in this study average time from injury to intervention was 52 hours.[23,24] Studies of spinal cord injury with intravenous steroids suggested that corticosteroids inhibited oxygen free radical–induced lipid peroxidation and decreased vasospasm. Findings from the National Acute Spinal Cord Injury Studies suggested that methylprednisolone given as a bolus of 30 mg/kg intravenously within 8 hours of injury, followed by 5.4 mg/kg/h for 23 to 48 hours, may be associated with improved neurologic function.[25] However, there have been significant side effects attributed to this steroid dose,[26] and a similar study, the Corticosteroid After Significant Head injury (CRASH) trial, showed an increased risk of death with megadose steroids after head injury.[27] Although these study results cannot be directly translated into the setting of isolated orbital trauma, megadose steroids cannot be recommended in an evidence-based fashion for TON, especially in patients with significant head injury given these increased systemic risks from the CRASH study.

As for surgical intervention, anecdotal reports have suggested potential improvement in vascular perfusion, but the International Optic Nerve Trauma Study did not show a benefit of optic canal decompression surgery.[20] One exception for which optic canal decompression might be considered is in the rare case where the bony canal is disrupted.

In summary, based on the existing literature, neither corticosteroids nor optic canal surgery should be considered standard of care for patients with TON. Clinicians must use their judgment to decide how to treat an individual patient.

ORBITAL TRAUMA–RELATED MOTILITY DISORDERS

Ocular misalignment, impaired extraocular motility, and pain on eye movement are often encountered after orbital fracture and may be the result of muscle contusion, malposition, or entrapment, cranial nerve palsy, mass effect of soft tissue edema or hemorrhage, and globe malposition. The clinician's initial task is to determine which patients require urgent surgery. Most often the impaired motility/alignment following fracture results from soft tissue edema and hemorrhage, is self-limited, and requires no intervention. Muscle entrapment, on the other hand, may require urgent surgical repair.

Clinically, the presence of restricted motility plus oculocardiac reflex (pain, bradycardia, and nausea on attempted eye movement) is highly suspicious for entrapment.[28] Entrapped muscles will usually cause greatest impaired motility in their field of action as well as restriction in the opposite direction (**Fig. 4**). Forced duction testing can be helpful, especially when patients cannot cooperate well on examination, although distinguishing a firm stop of entrapment versus a diffuse restriction from edema can be challenging. Generalized restriction in all directions, or a frozen globe, is concerning for orbital compartment syndrome.

Subacute motility and alignment deficits may evolve as enophthalmos develops and become more apparent when the initial periorbital edema resolves. Delayed fracture repair may be technically more challenging, so for larger fractures with significant tissue displacement likely to cause a motility disturbance or misalignment, repair within a week or 2 of injury may be preferable. The routine use of steroids in patients with orbital fractures is controversial. There are limited data suggesting that better outcomes in motility are achieved with their use.[29] Steroids do have the benefit of more rapid resolution of pain and swelling, which may be helpful not only in terms of patient comfort but also in allowing for more readily determining the cause of

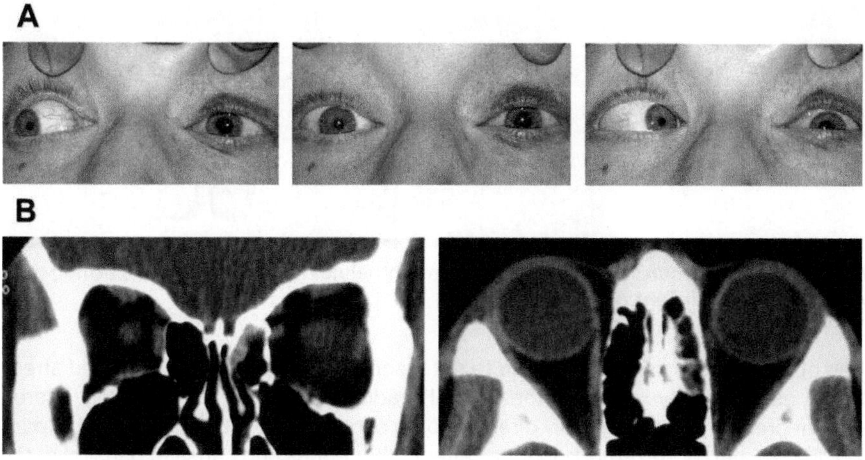

Fig. 4. Medial trapdoor fracture showing (*A*) restricted horizontal eye movements on the left side and (*B*) subtle findings of medial rectus asymmetry despite intact appearing medial well on CT, initially misread as normal. (*From* Yoon MK, McCulley TJ. Orbital disease in neuro-ophthalmology. Neurol Clin 2010;28(3):679–99.)

abnormal motility. Oral antibiotics are sometimes prescribed, especially if the orbit has been exposed to sinus contents.

ENOPHTHALMOS

Enophthalmos most commonly results from orbital fractures. However, in the absence of trauma, the differential for enophthalmos includes silent sinus syndrome, intracranial hypotension, metastatic scirrhous breast carcinoma, Parry-Romberg syndrome, linear scleroderma, lupus erythematosus profundus, and other rare inflammatory diseases.[30] Parry-Romberg syndrome is a phakomatosis also known as progressive hemifacial atrophy syndrome, which is often diagnosed in the first or second decade of life and is associated with epilepsy. Scleroderma is another rare disease characterized by localized fibrosis that may affect the growth of bones and soft tissue.

The term "silent sinus syndrome" was coined in 1994 by Soparkar and colleagues[31] and refers to spontaneous maxillary sinus atelectasis with orbital floor retraction and resorption causing ipsilateral enophthalmos and hypoglobus. Most often there are no sinus disease symptoms, and instead, patients present with globe displacement, and less commonly, with diplopia.[32–34] This syndrome may affect patients of all ages, with most commonly reported onset in the fourth decade of life.[35–39] The mechanism of maxillary atelectasis is postulated to be negative sinus pressure created by prolonged sinus hypoventilation due to outflow obstruction, and/or chronic inflammation with contraction of fibrous bands, resulting in distortion of the antral wall. In addition, bone resorption and remodeling contribute to orbital floor displacement and altered globe position (**Fig. 5**).[40,41]

Chronic intracranial hypotension has more recently been recognized to cause similar bony remodeling of the sinuses and orbits in what has been called the "sunken eyes, sagging brain syndrome."[42] Abnormally low intracranial pressure (ICP), most commonly from excessive cerebrospinal fluid shunting, exerts a pressure gradient on the bones of the skull that can lead to expanded orbital volume and subsequent enophthalmos. Specifically, low ICP can change the pressure gradient across the

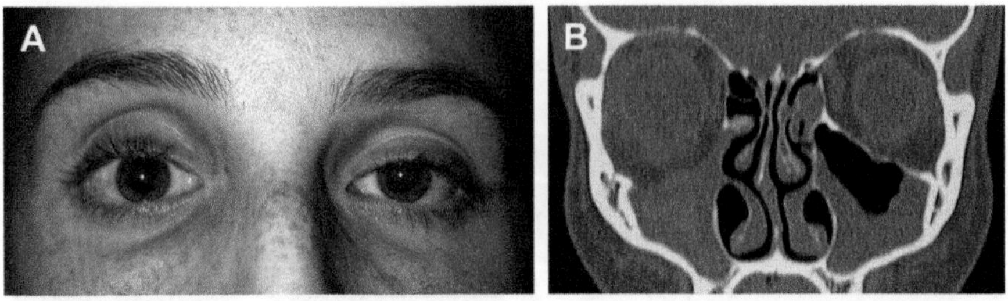

Fig. 5. Silent sinus syndrome clinically shows enophthalmos (*A*) and CT shows opacified sinus with remodeling of right orbital floor (*B*).

bone of the orbital roof and may lead to net resorption of bone from decreased stress as well as effectively reversing the normal gradient. It is theorized that this altered gradient creates an intracranially directed force across the roof causing orbital expansion. ICP-related bone remodeling may affect other bones and cause expansion of the sphenoid sinus (**Fig. 6**).[43,44] This radiographic sign may be useful in identifying patients with low ICP, who are at risk for related orbital disease.

In addition to cosmetic disfigurement, advanced disease can be vision threatening. As the enophthalmos progresses, a pocket of air forms in the space between the eyelid and the globe beneath the superior orbital rim, such that with supraduction, the cornea completely loses contact with the eyelid (**Fig. 7**). Several patients also develop optic neuropathy, likely relating to bony changes at the level of the orbit apex affecting the size and shape of the optic canals.[43]

Intracranial hypotension may also cause significant ocular motility problems by altering the relative position of the globe and muscles. Supraduction is particularly reduced due to the mechanical effect of the superior bowing of the orbital roof and displacement of the superior rectus muscle, analogous to the inferior rectus muscle displacement through a comminuted orbital floor fracture.[44] Abnormal horizontal ductions are less straightforward and may relate to shortening of the muscles with loss of optimal sarcomere filament overlap. Cranial nerve or brainstem abnormality may also contribute to impaired motility.

Initial management of sagging brain, sunken eyes syndrome should include correcting the intracranial hypotension.[42] ICP normalization will likely halt disease progression, and some patients may experience a small immediate reduction of enophthalmos, likely due to soft tissue and vascular changes.[42] If silent sinus syndrome is analogous, bony remodeling may occur spontaneously once the pressure

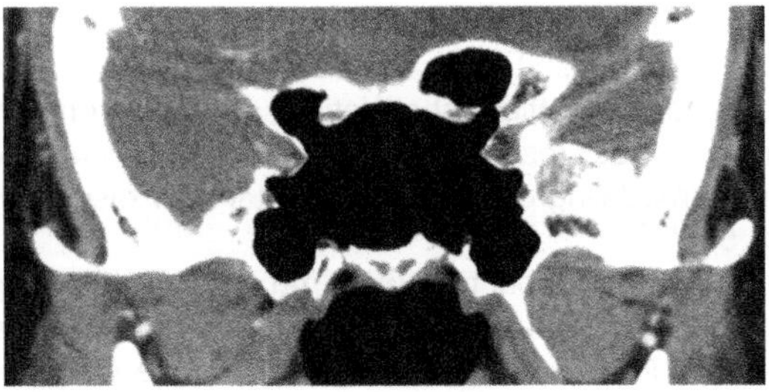

Fig. 6. Enlargement and "bubbling" of the sphenoid sinus is a sign of advanced chronic intracranial hypotension. (*From* McCulley TJ, Jordan Piluek W, Chang J. Intracranial pressure and skull remodeling. Saudi J Ophthalmol 2015;29(1):57–62.)

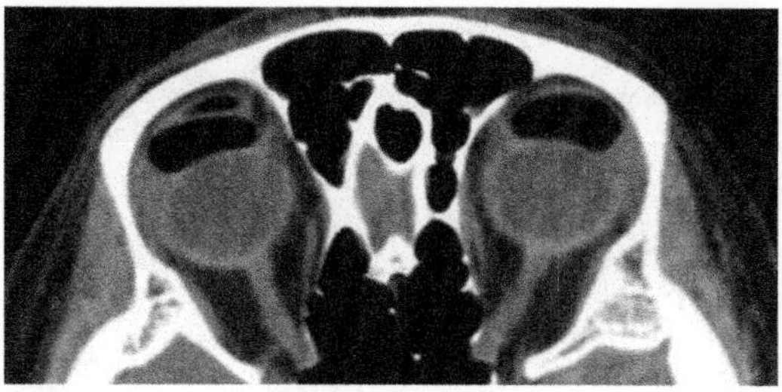

Fig. 7. Intracranial hypotension can lead to vision-threatening and disfiguring enophthalmos—note the air pockets between the globes and the orbital rim. (*From* McCulley TJ, Jordan Piluek W, Chang J. Intracranial pressure and skull remodeling. Saudi J Ophthalmol 2015; 29(1):57–62.)

gradient is normalized. In a series of 23 patients with silent sinus syndrome, 22 patients had partial or complete normalization of globe position after normalizing the aeration of the maxillary sinus.[41] Observation should therefore be considered following normalization of ICP before proceeding with surgical augmentation of the orbit. When medically necessary or when improvement is not seen following normalization of ICP, surgical intervention may be considered to augment orbital soft tissue volume with orbital floor and/or roof implants.[45–47] Patients with significant ocular surface disease may benefit from tarsorrhaphy, especially if they are unable or unwilling to undergo shunt revision or orbital surgery.

INFLAMMATION

There are numerous systemic diseases that can be associated with orbital inflammation, and proper history, examination, and workup should be pursued to evaluate for these. A thorough history is the first step in evaluating a patient with an inflamed orbit. A relatively short duration of hours to days favors infection. In contrast, a subacute presentation of days to weeks is more characteristic of TED or a neoplastic process. Any history of rheumatologic disease that might be associated with soft tissue inflammation, such as systemic lupus erythematosus (SLE) or polyarteritis nodosa, should be noted as well as a history of thyroid abnormalities. History of trauma or insect bites (risk factors for infection) and compromised immune status, for example, due to diabetes, may further point toward infection. The age of the patient is also key; because of their immature immune system, children are more apt to suffer from an infection, whereas the elderly are more likely to develop lymphoma.

It is important to note the position of the eyelid; most infectious and inflammatory conditions result in blepharoptosis or no change in the eyelid position, whereas TED causes retraction of the eyelid (**Fig. 8**). Nontender swelling and mild discomfort are more concerning for neoplasm or specific inflammatory syndromes such as granulomatosis with polyangiitis (GPA; formerly known as Wegener granulomatosis), whereas severe pain is more suggestive of myositis or orbital cellulitis.[48]

Workup of orbital inflammation inevitably requires orbital imaging. Most orbital surgeons prefer CT, which in most cases is an adequate first step. However, MRI provides much more soft tissue detail (**Fig. 9**) and can be used in conjunction with CT. Looking for signs of sinusitis is key: although the presence of sinusitis suggests infection, its absence increases the likelihood of idiopathic orbital inflammatory syndrome (IOIS), although difficulty arises with conditions such as GPA, which may affect the orbit and sinus simultaneously.

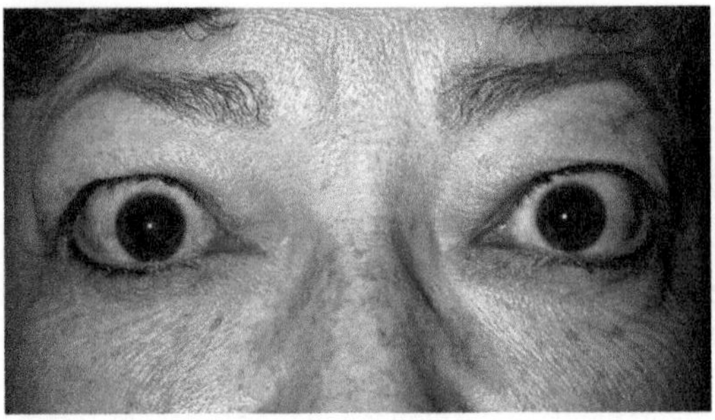

Fig. 8. TED shows eyelid retraction with lateral flare.

IDIOPATHIC ORBITAL INFLAMMATION

When the cause of an inflamed orbit cannot be determined, the term IOIS is applied. Formerly referred to as orbital pseudotumor, IOIS is a diagnosis of exclusion. Virtually any neuro-ophthalmic clinical feature can be mimicked by IOIS, depending on the site of inflammation.

When inflammation is centered primarily within a muscle, the term myositis is used. Myositis is apt to present to the neurologist, because it causes painful diplopia.[49] The pattern of misalignment can be that of paresis, restriction, or both. Inflammation of the lacrimal gland is called dacryoadenitis. Optic perineuritis refers to inflammation around the optic nerve sheath (as opposed to optic neuritis, which is inflammation of the nerve itself).[50] Tolosa-Hunt syndrome denotes idiopathic inflammation of the orbital apex and/or the cavernous sinus.[51] IOIS often involves more than one structure.

Focal inflammation within the orbit is typical of IOIS, presenting as swelling of one or more structures, such as the lacrimal gland, an extraocular muscle, or perineural tissue. When it is not possible to definitively distinguish an infection from IOIS in a patient with an acutely inflamed orbit, a diagnostic trial with antibiotics may be helpful. Infectious orbititis can carry grave consequences if misdiagnosed. Rhino-orbital-cerebral mucormycosis in particular constitutes a life-threatening emergency and should be suspected in immune-suppressed patients, particularly in those with poorly controlled diabetes (**Fig. 10**).[17]

In more clear-cut IOIS, treatment with steroids usually results in rapid resolution. The lack of rapid and complete resolution suggests alternative causes. A starting dose of 1 mg/kg prednisone, tapered over the course of 1 to 2 months following normalization, is a standard regimen. In recurrent or unresponsive disease, a systemic evaluation is appropriate. Laboratory testing for diseases listed in **Table 2** is

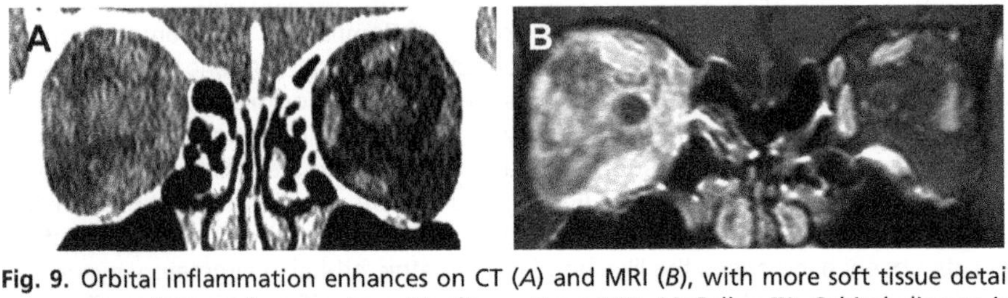

Fig. 9. Orbital inflammation enhances on CT (*A*) and MRI (*B*), with more soft tissue detail apparent on MRI, such as perineuritis. (*From* Yoon MK, McCulley TJ. Orbital disease in neuro-ophthalmology. Neurol Clin 2010;28(3):679–99.)

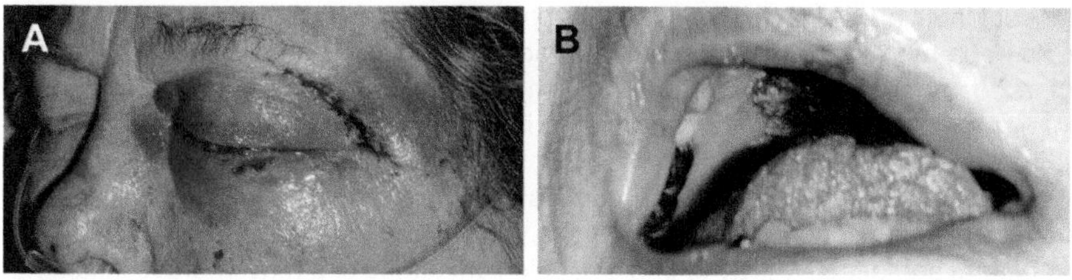

Fig. 10. (A) Mucormycosis of the orbit; (*B*) note the necrotic tissue in the palate. (*From* Yoon MK, McCulley TJ. Orbital disease in neuro-ophthalmology. Neurol Clin 2010;28(3):679–99.)

appropriate; assistance from rheumatology may be helpful. A CT chest scan may be helpful if the suspicion for sarcoidosis is high.

An orbital biopsy should be performed with atypical, recurrent, or steroid-unresponsive disease. If the diagnosis remains IOIS, the steroid dose can be increased and the duration of the taper lengthened. In cases refractory to steroids, more potent immune suppressive agents such as methotrexate or rituximab can be considered.[52,53] Radiation therapy can also be used in select cases; however, results are variable and often unsatisfactory.[54,55]

THYROID EYE DISEASE

Approximately 50% of patients with Graves disease will develop TED. The progressive (active) inflammatory phase of TED is characterized by orbital discomfort, periocular

Table 2
Differential diagnosis for orbital inflammation

Infectious	Bacterial	*Staphylococcus aureus* *Streptococcus pyogenes*
	Fungal	Mucormycosis Aspergillosis
	Parasitic	Cysticercosis Trichinosis Microfilaria Echinococcus
	Viral	Epstein-Barr virus (eg, dacryoadenitis) Varicella zoster virus (herpes zoster ophthalmicus)
Systemic inflammatory syndromes	Vasculitis	GPA Polyarteritis nodosa Rheumatoid arthritis Hepatitis-related vasculitis Relapsing polychondritis
	Miscellaneous	TED Sarcoidosis IgG4-RD SLE
Neoplastic		Lymphoma Rhabdomyosarcoma Ruptured dermoid cyst
Vascular		Carotid-cavernous fistula Orbital lymphatic malformation (lymphangioma)
No identifiable cause		IOIS

and conjunctival edema and redness, and progression in proptosis, strabismus, or optic neuropathy. In contrast to myositis, extraocular muscle enlargement in TED is characterized by sparing of the tendon, which may be a useful sign on CT and MRI. Controlling the patient's endocrine status is essential but does not usually reverse the orbitopathy. Smoking cessation should be encouraged in all patients. Correcting selenium deficiency has also been suggested to aid thyroid function normalization and may also impact orbital manifestations.[56] Consumption of only 2 Brazil nuts daily is a natural and effective way to improve selenium status and may improve inflammatory markers overexpressed in orbital tissue in TED, such as interleukin-1 (IL-1), IL-6, tumor necrosis factor-α, and interferon-γ levels.[57,58]

Urgent treatment is required for proptosis severe enough to cause lagophthalmos, exposure keratopathy, or signs of compressive optic neuropathy in TED. Optic neuropathy is often accompanied by restricted eye movements and is usually related to apical crowding with enlarged extraocular muscles on imaging. Steroid pulse therapy with intravenous methylprednisolone (500–1000 mg weekly for 6 weeks) is more effective and carries fewer side effects than 1 mg/kg oral prednisone. If there is no response to steroids, urgent orbital decompression is required for vision-threatening conditions. Steroid-sparing and disease-specific therapies are being investigated, including rituximab, tocilizumab, adalimumab, teprotumumab, and other agents, such as druglike small-molecule TSHR antagonists.[59]

SARCOIDOSIS

Sarcoidosis may affect one or many organs throughout the body and has a highly variable presentation in the orbit as well.[60] Sarcoidosis should be suspected and worked up when relatively nontender inflammation of the lacrimal glands is encountered, particularly in patients of African descent. The lacrimal gland is the most common site of involvement, in 42% to 63% of patients, followed by orbit, eyelid, and lacrimal sac.[61,62] Diagnosis can be made by conjunctival and/or lacrimal gland biopsy. Treatment involves steroids and sometimes methotrexate or other immunosuppressive medications.

IgG4-RELATED ORBITAL DISEASE

Lymphoproliferative disease encompasses a wide spectrum between reactive inflammatory disease and lymphoma. More recently, a subtype enriched with plasma cells expressing IgG4 has come to attention.[63] Similar to sarcoidosis, IgG4-related disease (IgG4-RD) is a great mimicker and affects different organs. About half of all orbital cases are associated with systemic disease, and it seems likely that many cases previously labeled as IOIS actually constitute IgG4-RD.[64,65] The epidemiology is still poorly defined. The largest series of patients come from Japan, where the disease was first described.[66] Average patients are middle aged, and orbital disease affects men and women equally. Several patterns of orbital involvement have been described: sclerosing dacryoadenitis, myositis with nerve enlargement (most commonly the infraorbital nerve), often in combination with sinus disease, eosinophilia, pachymeningitis, systemic involvement, and sclerosing orbital inflammation (**Fig. 11**).[67] Current consensus for diagnostic criteria on pathology includes a dense lymphoplasmacytic infiltrate with elevated IgG4+/IgG+ plasma cell ratio, storiform fibrosis, and obliterative phlebitis.[68] Serum IgG4 may or may not be elevated. The disease is usually treated with steroids but may require other agents such as methotrexate or rituximab.[69] Like other chronic inflammatory disorders (eg, TED), IgG4-RD is probably associated with an increased risk of lymphoma.[70]

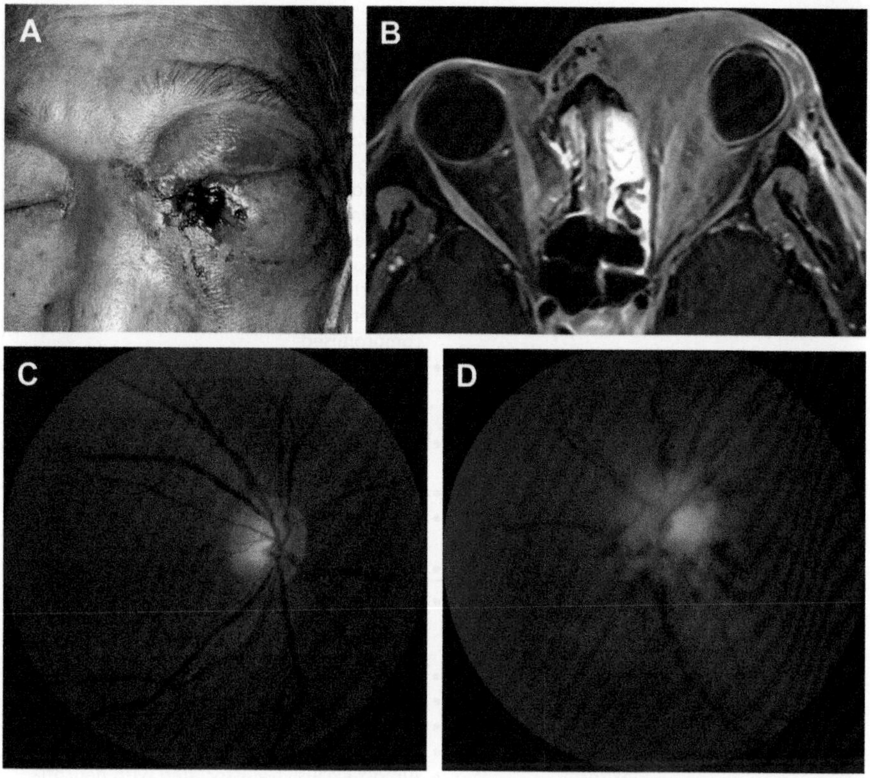

Fig. 11. A severe presentation of IgG4-related orbital disease (*A*) with MRI (*B*) and fundus photos of the right (*C*) and left eyes (*D*).

NEOPLASTIC

Orbital neoplasm may give rise to virtually any neuro-ophthalmic symptom or sign. Any extraocular muscle or cranial nerve passing through the orbit can be affected. Ocular misalignment and diplopia in the setting of neoplasia can result from direct involvement of one or more cranial nerves or muscles, or indirectly from mass effect. Optic neuropathy occurs from compression with larger or apical tumors as well as from intrinsic tumors of the optic nerve (eg, glioma) or its sheath (eg, meningioma). **Table 3** highlights common orbital neoplasms in children and adults and key clinical features.

The most common benign primary tumors of adults are cavernous hemangiomas, and in children, are capillary hemangiomas and dermoids. Lymphoma is the most common malignant primary orbital tumors in adults, followed by lacrimal gland tumors, whereas in children, the most common malignant primary malignant tumor is rhabdomyosarcoma.[71]

Metastases comprise a significant portion of orbital malignancies in both children and adults. Twenty percent of children with neuroblastoma develop orbital involvement, which characteristically gives rise to unilateral or bilateral proptosis and nontraumatic periorbital ecchymosis.[72] In adults, the most frequent primary sites for orbital metastases are breast, kidney, lung, and skin.[73]

Table 3
Neoplasms of the orbit

Category	Specific Neoplasm	Clinical Pearls
Vascular	Cavernous hemangioma	• Most common benign orbital tumor in adults • Usually intraconal, slow-growing • Presents with proptosis, may be incidental finding
	Capillary hemangioma	• Most common benign orbital tumor in children • Enlarges in first 1–2 y of life, then involutes • Amblyopia may occur (multiple mechanisms, eg, occlusive, refractive) • Intervention indicated when vision is compromised • Treated with β-blockers (systemic or topical) or steroids (systemic or intralesional injection)
	Lymphatic malformation (also called lymphangioma)	• Benign tumor of lymphatics and variable other vascular components • Features may overlap with orbital varix • Spontaneous hemorrhage may occur (chocolate cyst) • May enlarge with systemic infections
Neural	Meningioma	• Most common optic nerve tumor in adults; may arise from optic nerve sheath, periorbita, or extend to orbit from intracranial origin • More common in women
	Glioma	• Most common optic nerve tumor in children • Usually benign • Often associated with neurofibromatosis 1
	Plexiform neurofibroma	• Almost exclusively associated with neurofibromatosis type I • Diffusely infiltrative, often with intracranial involvement
	Schwannoma	• Benign tumor of Schwann cells, often arising from supraorbital nerve • May have intracranial component limiting complete excision
Mesenchymal	Rhabdomyosarcoma	• Most common primary orbital malignancy in children • May present with rapid onset of symptoms resembling cellulitis • Responsive to radiation treatment and chemotherapy
	Osteoma	• Benign well-circumscribed bony tumor with radiolucent center • Often originates in frontal or ethmoid bone
	Fibrous dysplasia	• Usually presents in childhood and may stabilize with skeletal maturation • Bone replaced by fibrous-osseous tissue, may cause optic canal stenosis • Occurs in McCune Albright syndrome
	Osteosarcoma, chondrosarcoma	• Rare malignant tumors • Osteosarcoma may be associated with retinoblastoma especially after prior radiation treatment

(*continued on next page*)

Table 3
(*continued*)

Category	Specific Neoplasm	Clinical Pearls
Lacrimal	Pleomorphic adenoma	• Most common benign lacrimal gland neoplasm, presents with several years of gradual globe dystopia • Excise completely—incisional biopsy may increase risk of malignant transformation
	Adenoid cystic carcinoma	• Most common malignant epithelial tumor of the lacrimal gland • Presents with pain (perineural spread)
Cutaneous	Dermoid cyst	• Common benign congenital tumor, often detected in first 2 y of life but rarely presents in adulthood • Most often found at frontozygomatic suture, sometimes with "dumbbell" configuration, sometimes entirely within orbit • Rupture incites inflammatory response
	SCC	• Often extends to orbit via perineural spread • Consider in patients with history of previously excised periocular SCC
	BCC	• Usually from neglected or incompletely excised periocular BCC
Lymphoproliferative	Lymphoma	• Most common form of orbital lymphoproliferative lesion is MALT (mucosal associated lymphoid tissue) lymphoma • May involve multiple orbital structures, has predilection for lacrimal gland • May be bilateral • May be associated with systemic disease
Metastatic disease	Breast cancer	• Most common metastasis to orbit in women
	Lung cancer	• Most common metastasis to orbit in men
	Neuroblastoma	• Most common metastasis to orbit in children • May give rise to periocular ecchymoses ("raccoon eye")
Secondary invasion	Sinus	• Mucocele from frontal or ethmoidal sinuses • Sinus carcinomas carry poor prognosis

Globe malposition in the absence of significant pain or inflammation often provides an important clue in diagnosing an orbital neoplasm. The eye is expected to move opposite to the direction of the tumor, thus inferomedial displacement of the eye is seen with lacrimal gland tumors, and intraconal tumors usually create axial proptosis (**Fig. 12**). Most orbital tumors will cause some globe malposition before reaching substantial enough size to cause nerve compression, except at the apex, where even a relatively small tumor may compress nerves before the development of globe malposition. Optic nerve edema is seen when optic nerve compression is within 1 cm of the globe; otherwise, one may only see pallor from chronic posterior compression. Choroidal folds may be seen when the globe itself is compressed.

Another pattern of orbital neoplastic disease presentation relates to neoplasms with a tendency for perineural spread; squamous cell carcinoma (SSC) and adenoid cystic carcinoma are known for this property but even basal cell carcinoma (BCC) can manifest in this way. Orbital involvement may present with periorbital pain, numbness, or cranial neuropathies rather than a significant mass effect. Although direct extension of

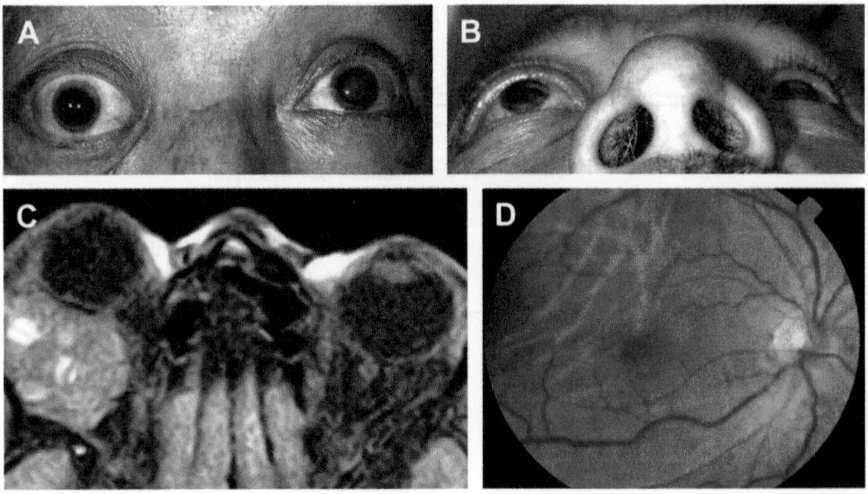

Fig. 12. Inferomedial globe malposition (*A*) and proptosis (*B*) from a lacrimal gland lesion (in this case adenocystic carcinoma), with MRI (*C*) and fundus findings (*D*: choroidal folds). (*From* Yoon MK, McCulley TJ. Orbital disease in neuro-ophthalmology. Neurol Clin 2010; 28(3):679–99.)

such local tumors is often clinically obvious, the diagnosis can be very challenging when patients present long after (incomplete) excision of the primary facial skin lesion.[74,75]

Whenever an intraorbital tumor is suspected, imaging is mandatory. MRI is most sensitive for soft tissue involvement and hence the ideal modality in most circumstances. CT remains the preferred technique when assessment of bone is needed. Individualized treatment and follow-up vary with disease cause and often requires a multidisciplinary approach. All malignant tumors warrant evaluation by oncology, and tumors with intracranial or sinus extension should be evaluated by neurosurgery or otolaryngology, respectively. Benign tumors are usually amenable to complete excision, whereas malignant tumors often require a more complex approach, including radiation and/or chemotherapy.

REFERENCES

1. Boyette JR, Pemberton JD, Bonilla-Velez J. Management of orbital fractures: challenges and solutions. Clin Ophthalmol 2015;9:2127–37.
2. Kum C, McCulley TJ, Yoon MK, et al. Adult orbital trapdoor fracture. Ophthal Plast Reconstr Surg 2009;25(6):486–7.
3. McCulley TJ, Yip CC, Kersten RC, et al. Medial rectus muscle incarceration in pediatric medial orbital wall trapdoor fractures. Eur J Ophthalmol 2004;14(4):330–3.
4. Phan LT, Jordan Piluek W, McCulley TJ. Orbital trapdoor fractures. Saudi J Ophthalmol 2012;26(3):277–82.
5. Yip CC, McCulley TJ, Kersten RC, et al. Proptosis after hair pulling. Ophthal Plast Reconstr Surg 2003;19(2):154–5.
6. Elia MD, Shield D, Kazim M, et al. Spontaneous subperiosteal orbital hemorrhage. Orbit 2013;32(5):333–5.
7. Phan IT, Hoyt WF, McCulley TJ, et al. Blindness from orbital varices: case report. Orbit 2009;28(5):303–5.

8. Yoon MK, McCulley TJ. Non-traumatic subperiosteal orbital hematoma as a presenting sign of chronic myelogenous leukemia. Ophthal Plast Reconstr Surg 2012;28(4):e79–80.
9. Zoumalan CI, Bullock JD, Warwar RE, et al. Evaluation of intraocular and orbital pressure in the management of orbital hemorrhage: an experimental model. Arch Ophthalmol 2008;126(9):1257–60.
10. Schabdach DG, Goldberg SH, Breton ME, et al. An animal model of visual loss from orbital hemorrhage. Ophthal Plast Reconstr Surg 1994;10(3):200–5.
11. Otto AJ, Koornneef L, Mourits MP, et al. Retrobulbar pressures measured during surgical decompression of the orbit. Br J Ophthalmol 1996;80(12):1042–5.
12. Hargaden M, Goldberg SH, Cunningham D, et al. Optic neuropathy following simulation of orbital hemorrhage in the nonhuman primate. Ophthal Plast Reconstr Surg 1996;12(4):264–72.
13. Hayreh SS, Jonas JB. Optic disk and retinal nerve fiber layer damage after transient central retinal artery occlusion: an experimental study in rhesus monkeys. Am J Ophthalmol 2000;129(6):786–95.
14. Katz B, Herschler J, Brick DC. Orbital haemorrhage and prolonged blindness: a treatable posterior optic neuropathy. Br J Ophthalmol 1983;67(8):549–53.
15. Yoon MK, McCulley TJ. Orbital disease in neuro-ophthalmology. Neurol Clin 2010; 28(3):679–99.
16. Yu SS, Lee SH, Shin HW, et al. Traumatic carotid-cavernous sinus fistula in a patient with facial bone fractures. Arch Plast Surg 2015;42(6):791–3.
17. Lemos J, Eggenberger E. Neuro-ophthalmological emergencies. Neurohospitalist 2015;5(4):223–33.
18. Steinsapir KD, Goldberg RA. Traumatic optic neuropathy. Surv Ophthalmol 1994; 38(6):487–518.
19. Singman EL, Daphalapurkar N, White H, et al. Indirect traumatic optic neuropathy. Mil Med Res 2016;3:2.
20. Levin LA, Beck RW, Joseph MP, et al. The treatment of traumatic optic neuropathy: the International Optic Nerve Trauma Study. Ophthalmology 1999;106(7):1268–77.
21. Seiff SR. High dose corticosteroids for treatment of vision loss due to indirect injury to the optic nerve. Ophthalmic Surg 1990;21(6):389–95.
22. Anderson RL, Panje WR, Gross CE. Optic nerve blindness following blunt forehead trauma. Ophthalmology 1982;89(5):445–55.
23. Entezari M, Rajavi Z, Sedighi N, et al. High-dose intravenous methylprednisolone in recent traumatic optic neuropathy; a randomized double-masked placebo-controlled clinical trial. Graefes Arch Clin Exp Ophthalmol 2007;245(9):1267–71.
24. Yu-Wai-Man P, Griffiths PG. Steroids for traumatic optic neuropathy. Cochrane Database Syst Rev 2013;6:CD006032. [indicates systematic reviews/meta-analyses].
25. Bracken MB. Steroids for acute spinal cord injury. Cochrane Database Syst Rev 2012;1:CD001046. [indicates systematic reviews/meta-analyses].
26. Lee HC, Cho DY, Lee WY, et al. Pitfalls in treatment of acute cervical spinal cord injury using high-dose methylprednisolone: a retrospect audit of 111 patients. Surg Neurol 2007;68(Suppl 1):S37–41 [discussion: S41–2].
27. Edwards P, Arango M, Balica L, et al. Final results of MRC CRASH, a randomised placebo-controlled trial of intravenous corticosteroid in adults with head injury-outcomes at 6 months. Lancet 2005;365(9475):1957–9.
28. Swamy L, Phan LT, Sadah ZM, et al. Oculocardiac reflex in a medial orbital wall fracture without clinically evident entrapment. Middle East Afr J Ophthalmol 2013; 20(3):268–70.

29. Millman AL, Della Rocca RC, Spector S, et al. Steroids and orbital blowout fractures–a new systematic concept in medical management and surgical decision-making. Adv Ophthalmic Plast Reconstr Surg 1987;6:291–300.
30. Kao TY, Yoon MK, McCulley TJ, et al. Acquired enophthalmos in lupus erythematosus profundus. J Neuroophthalmol 2010;30(1):64–6.
31. Soparkar CN, Patrinely JR, Cuaycong MJ, et al. The silent sinus syndrome. A cause of spontaneous enophthalmos. Ophthalmology 1994;101(4):772–8.
32. Borruat FX, Jaques B, Durig J. Transient vertical diplopia and silent sinus disorder. J Neuroophthalmol 1999;19(3):173–5.
33. Wan MK, Francis IC, Carter PR, et al. The spectrum of presentation of silent sinus syndrome. J Neuroophthalmol 2000;20(3):207–12.
34. Yip CC, McCulley TJ, Kersten RC, et al. Silent sinus syndrome as a cause of diplopia in a child. J Pediatr Ophthalmol Strabismus 2003;40(5):309–11.
35. Davidson JK, Soparkar CN, Williams JB, et al. Negative sinus pressure and normal predisease imaging in silent sinus syndrome. Arch Ophthalmol 1999; 117(12):1653–4.
36. Gillman GS, Schaitkin BM, May M. Asymptomatic enophthalmos: the silent sinus syndrome. Am J Rhinol 1999;13(6):459–62.
37. Hunt SM, Tami TA. Sinusitis-induced enophthalmos: the silent sinus syndrome. Ear Nose Throat J 2000;79(8):576, 579–81, 584.
38. Rose TP. Spontaneous enophthalmos associated with asymptomatic maxillary sinus disease (silent sinus syndrome): case report. J Am Optom Assoc 1998;69(4): 236–40.
39. Vander Meer JB, Harris G, Toohill RJ, et al. The silent sinus syndrome: a case series and literature review. Laryngoscope 2001;111(6):975–8.
40. Rose GE, Sandy C, Hallberg L, et al. Clinical and radiologic characteristics of the imploding antrum, or "silent sinus," syndrome. Ophthalmology 2003;110(4): 811–8.
41. Sivasubramaniam R, Sacks R, Thornton M. Silent sinus syndrome: dynamic changes in the position of the orbital floor after restoration of normal sinus pressure. J Laryngol Otol 2011;125(12):1239–43.
42. Hwang TN, Rofagha S, McDermott MW, et al. Sunken eyes, sagging brain syndrome: bilateral enophthalmos from chronic intracranial hypotension. Ophthalmology 2011;118(11):2286–95.
43. McCulley TJ. Sphenoid sinus expansion: a radiographic sign of intracranial hypotension and the sunken eyes, sagging brain syndrome (an American Ophthalmological Society thesis). Trans Am Ophthalmol Soc 2013;111:145–54.
44. McCulley TJ, Jordan Piluek W, Chang J. Intracranial pressure and skull remodeling. Saudi J Ophthalmol 2015;29(1):57–62.
45. Bernardini FP, Rose GE, Cruz AA, et al. Gross enophthalmos after cerebrospinal fluid shunting for childhood hydrocephalus: the "silent brain syndrome". Ophthal Plast Reconstr Surg 2009;25(6):434–6.
46. Cruz AA, Mesquita IM, de Oliveira RS. Progressive bilateral enophthalmos associated with cerebrospinal shunting. Ophthal Plast Reconstr Surg 2008;24(2): 152–4.
47. Meyer DR, Nerad JA, Newman NJ, et al. Bilateral enophthalmos associated with hydrocephalus and ventriculoperitoneal shunting. Arch Ophthalmol 1996; 114(10):1206–9.
48. Bhatia A, Yadava U, Goyal JL, et al. Limited Wegener's granulomatosis of the orbit: a case study and review of literature. Eye (Lond) 2005;19(1):102–4.

49. Montagnese F, Wenninger S, Schoser B. "Orbiting around" the orbital myositis: clinical features, differential diagnosis and therapy. J Neurol 2016;263(4):631–40.
50. Pakdaman MN, Sepahdari AR, Elkhamary SM. Orbital inflammatory disease: pictorial review and differential diagnosis. World J Radiol 2014;6(4):106–15.
51. Smith JL, Taxdal DS. Painful ophthalmoplegia. The Tolosa-Hunt syndrome. Am J Ophthalmol 1966;61(6):1466–72.
52. Shah SS, Lowder CY, Schmitt MA, et al. Low-dose methotrexate therapy for ocular inflammatory disease. Ophthalmology 1992;99(9):1419–23.
53. Suhler EB, Lim LL, Beardsley RM, et al. Rituximab therapy for refractory orbital inflammation: results of a phase 1/2, dose-ranging, randomized clinical trial. JAMA Ophthalmol 2014;132(5):572–8.
54. Lee JH, Kim YS, Yang SW, et al. Radiotherapy with or without surgery for patients with idiopathic sclerosing orbital inflammation refractory or intolerant to steroid therapy. Int J Radiat Oncol Biol Phys 2012;84(1):52–8.
55. Smitt MC, Donaldson SS. Radiation therapy for benign disease of the orbit. Semin Radiat Oncol 1999;9(2):179–89.
56. Marcocci C, Kahaly GJ, Krassas GE, et al. Selenium and the course of mild Graves' orbitopathy. N Engl J Med 2011;364(20):1920–31.
57. Colpo E, Dalton DAVC, Reetz LG, et al. Brazilian nut consumption by healthy volunteers improves inflammatory parameters. Nutrition 2014;30(4):459–65.
58. Thomson CD, Chisholm A, McLachlan SK, et al. Brazil nuts: an effective way to improve selenium status. Am J Clin Nutr 2008;87(2):379–84.
59. Shan SJ, Douglas RS. The pathophysiology of thyroid eye disease. J Neuroophthalmol 2014;34(2):177–85.
60. Liu D, Birnbaum AD. Update on sarcoidosis. Curr Opin Ophthalmol 2015;26(6):512–6.
61. Demirci H, Christianson MD. Orbital and adnexal involvement in sarcoidosis: analysis of clinical features and systemic disease in 30 cases. Am J Ophthalmol 2011;151(6):1074–80.e1.
62. Prabhakaran VC, Saeed P, Esmaeli B, et al. Orbital and adnexal sarcoidosis. Arch Ophthalmol 2007;125(12):1657–62.
63. Stone JH, Zen Y, Deshpande V. IgG4-related disease. N Engl J Med 2012;366(6):539–51.
64. Wallace ZS, Khosroshahi A, Jakobiec FA, et al. IgG4-related systemic disease as a cause of "idiopathic" orbital inflammation, including orbital myositis, and trigeminal nerve involvement. Surv Ophthalmol 2012;57(1):26–33.
65. Wu A, Andrew NH, McNab AA, et al. IgG4-related ophthalmic disease: pooling of published cases and literature review. Curr Allergy Asthma Rep 2015;15(6):27.
66. Hamano H, Kawa S, Horiuchi A, et al. High serum IgG4 concentrations in patients with sclerosing pancreatitis. N Engl J Med 2001;344(10):732–8.
67. Wu A, Andrew NH, McNab AA, et al. Bilateral IgG4-related ophthalmic disease: a strong indication for systemic imaging. Br J Ophthalmol 2015. [Epub ahead of print].
68. Deshpande V, Zen Y, Chan JK, et al. Consensus statement on the pathology of IgG4-related disease. Mod Pathol 2012;25(9):1181–92.
69. Khosroshahi A, Carruthers MN, Deshpande V, et al. Rituximab for the treatment of IgG4-related disease: lessons from 10 consecutive patients. Medicine (Baltimore) 2012;91(1):57–66.
70. McNab AA, McKelvie P. IgG4-related ophthalmic disease. Part II: clinical aspects. Ophthal Plast Reconstr Surg 2015;31(3):167–78.

71. Koopman JH, van der Heiden-van der Loo M, van Dijk MR, et al. Incidence of primary malignant orbital tumours in the Netherlands. Eye (Lond) 2011;25(4):461–5.
72. Rao AA, Naheedy JH, Chen JY, et al. A clinical update and radiologic review of pediatric orbital and ocular tumors. J Oncol 2013;2013:975908.
73. Magliozzi P, Strianese D, Bonavolonta P, et al. Orbital metastases in Italy. Int J Ophthalmol 2015;8(5):1018–23.
74. Bowyer JD, Sullivan TJ, Whitehead KJ, et al. The management of perineural spread of squamous cell carcinoma to the ocular adnexae. Ophthal Plast Reconstr Surg 2003;19(4):275–81.
75. Clouston PD, Sharpe DM, Corbett AJ, et al. Perineural spread of cutaneous head and neck cancer. Its orbital and central neurologic complications. Arch Neurol 1990;47(1):73–7.

The Yield of Diagnostic Imaging in Patients with Isolated Horner Syndrome

Johanna D. Beebe, MD[a], Randy H. Kardon, MD, PhD[a,b,*], Matthew J. Thurtell, MBBS, MSc[a]

KEYWORDS

- Isolated Horner syndrome • Anisocoria • Imaging yield • Carotid artery dissection

KEY POINTS

- Patients with Horner syndrome (oculosympathetic defect) may be associated with signs and symptoms that help determine the cause and localization of the defect.
- Isolated Horner syndrome is defined as an oculosympathetic defect *without* associated signs and symptoms (except for pain) and it presents a diagnostic dilemma in which neuroimaging is indicated.
- Imaging of isolated Horner syndrome in a consecutive case series yielded a structural cause in 20% of patients with the most common cause being a carotid dissection.

INTRODUCTION

Horner syndrome is a clinical constellation of symptoms and signs classically including ipsilateral ptosis, pupillary miosis, and facial anhidrosis due to a lesion of the oculosympathetic pathway. The 3-neuron length of the oculosympathetic pathway produces a diagnostic challenge for the clinician with a patient who presents with a clinically isolated Horner syndrome.[1]

This work was supported in part by the Department of Veterans Affairs, Veterans Health Administration, Office of Research and Development, Rehabilitation Research and Development, and Iowa City VA Center of Excellence for the Prevention and Treatment of Visual Loss: C9251-C (R.H. Kardon), and an unrestricted grant from Research to Prevent Blindness (New York, NY).
Disclosures: R.H. Kardon is a consultant for Novartis (Steering Committee for OCTiMS Multicenter study on OCT over time in MS patients). He is also a cofounder of MedFace LLC and FaceX LLC.
[a] Department of Ophthalmology and Visual Sciences, University of Iowa Hospital and Clinics, 200 Hawkins Drive, Iowa City, IA 52242, USA; [b] Iowa City Veterans Affairs Medical Center, Highway 6, Iowa City, IA 52246, USA
* Corresponding author. Department of Ophthalmology and Visual Sciences, University of Iowa Hospitals and Clinics, 11290D PFP, 200 Hawkins Drive, Iowa City, IA 52242.
E-mail address: randy-kardon@uiowa.edu

Neurol Clin 35 (2017) 145–151
http://dx.doi.org/10.1016/j.ncl.2016.08.005
0733-8619/17/Published by Elsevier Inc.

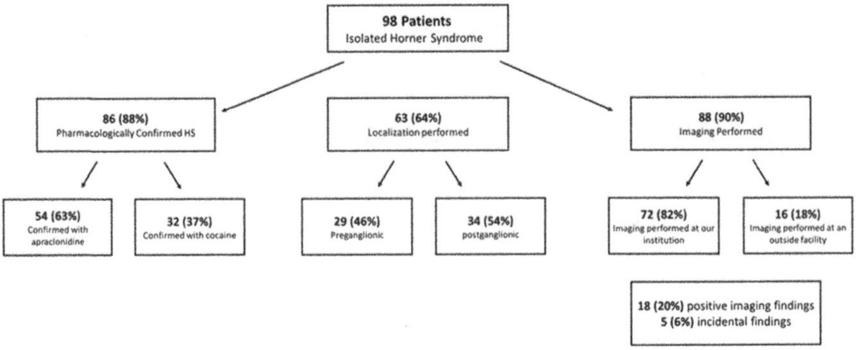

Fig. 1. The distribution of the testing, localization, and imaging yield of the 98 patients with isolated Horner syndrome (HS).

Determining the cause of Horner syndrome is justified, because a sinister underlying condition could be present, in which the patient would benefit from early diagnosis. Topical pharmacologic testing with apraclonidine or cocaine can be used to diagnose Horner syndrome or it may be determined clinically.[2] Hydroxyamphetamine pharmacologic testing can be used to localize the oculosympathetic lesion as being preganglionic (first-order or second-order neuron lesion) or postganglionic (third-order neuron lesion),[3] but it now has limited availability. Some clinicians use pharmacologic testing to help focus the interpretation of subsequent imaging.[4] There are a number of studies that advocate for a systematic approach to localization of the lesion using associated signs and symptoms, and then performing subsequent anatomically focused imaging with either MRI or computed tomography (CT) with angiography. For example, Reede and colleagues[2] advocate for identifying whether the Horner syndrome is a first-order, second-order, or third-order neuron lesion and performing focused imaging with either CT or MRI. Digre and colleagues[5] separated patients based on preganglionic and postganglionic lesions with pharmacologic testing or clinical localization, and imaged this select region. Davagnanam and colleagues[4] developed an imaging algorithm separating patients with first-order neuron lesions from those with second-order and third-order neuron lesions. In this algorithm, first-order neuron lesions were imaged with MRI, including the brain, cervical spinal cord, and upper thoracic spinal cord. Second-order and third-order neuron lesions were imaged with CT angiography from the orbits to T4 to T5. Davagnanam and colleagues[4] touched on the challenges of approaching patients with clinically isolated Horner syndrome, suggesting that these patients would be best evaluated within 6 weeks. However, they do not recommend specific imaging modalities, but rather that the study type be chosen at the clinician's discretion. Of note, the investigators defined isolated Horner syndrome to include patients who lack localizing signs, but also did not have a personal history of malignancy or pain.

Our study was motivated by the clinical conundrum presented by isolated Horner syndrome, as these patients do not lend themselves to decision trees of traditional neurologic localization and have a wide variety of potentially sinister causes. We defined a patient to have an isolated Horner syndrome if the patient presented without other clinical signs to aid in localization following a thorough history and physical examination. For this study, patients with pain or headache were not excluded and could be considered to have isolated Horner syndrome. Ultimately, we sought to determine the yield of imaging in this population and to identify the most common causes for this often subtle, isolated syndrome.

METHODS

We conducted a retrospective chart review of patients who were coded as having Horner syndrome after being seen in the University of Iowa Neuro-Ophthalmology Clinic between 2000 and 2014. Patients in whom the diagnosis of Horner syndrome could be confidently made clinically were included, and the method of those tested pharmacologically was recorded. Additionally, it was also noted if the patient's Horner syndrome was isolated or part of constellation of symptoms that would lend to localization. Those patients with localizing signs were ultimately excluded from this study, because they were not considered as having an isolated Horner syndrome. Symptoms of pain or headache were not considered to be a localizing factor and those patients were included as having isolated Horner syndrome. In review of the cases, it was noted whether the patient underwent imaging at an outside facility or at the University of Iowa Hospitals and Clinics. All patients in whom imaging was obtained at the University of Iowa underwent a specified Horner imaging protocol, unless contraindicated. This protocol involved obtaining an MRI/magnetic resonance angiography (MRA) of the oculosympathetic pathway from the supraorbital ridge to T4 with fat suppression and postcontrast images. Outside images were reviewed by a neuro-ophthalmologist. It was noted whether the Horner syndrome was judged to be acquired or potentially congenital, based on history or examination. Patients with congenital Horner syndrome were excluded from this analysis. Demographic characteristics were also recorded. Additionally, we report the incidental imaging findings in these patients, which often required additional workup.

RESULTS

Our retrospective review identified 98 patients with clinically isolated Horner syndrome; 50 men and 48 women with an average age of 54 years (**Fig. 1**). Of the 98 patients with isolated Horner syndrome, 86 underwent pharmacologic testing to

Table 1
The diagnosis of the 18 patients with identifiable causes of isolated Horner syndrome

Cause of Isolated Horner Syndrome	n
Carotid artery dissection	7
C5–C6 disc osteophyte	1
Carotid artery sheath mass, biopsy consistent with sarcoidosis	1
Vertebral artery dissection following chiropractic manipulation	1
Prominent bilateral cervical lymph nodes; extensive workup with hematology/oncology, determined to be reactive	1
C5–C6 cervical disc herniation	1
Fungal intracavitary apical lung lesion	1
Chiari malformation with syringobulbia and syringomyelia	1
C7–T1 perineural cyst	1
T1 paraspinal lesion and lymphadenopathy, and apical lung disease; all due to progression of known metastatic breast cancer	1
Left supraclinoid internal carotid aneurysm	1
Extranodal marginal zone B-cell lymphoma of the right orbit	1

Table 2
The pharmacologic testing and localization for the patients who underwent further workup for incidental imaging findings

n	Pharmacologically Confirmed Horner Syndrome	Hydroxyamphetamine Localization	Incidental Finding with Final Diagnosis
1	Apraclonidine 0.5%	Preganglionic Left Horner	Benign left thyroid cyst (<5 mm)
2	Apraclonidine 0.5%	Postganglionic Left Horner	Cystic small pituitary adenoma not involving cavernous sinus
3	Apraclonidine 0.5%	Preganglionic Right Horner	Left 0.5 cm frontal meningioma
4	Cocaine 10%	None performed Right Horner	Large left posterior fossa developmental venous anomaly
5	Apraclonidine 0.5%	Postganglionic	Parotid gland basaloid neoplasm

confirm the diagnosis, whereas 12 patients had unequivocal signs of Horner syndrome not requiring pharmacologic testing. Apraclonidine 0.5% was used in 54 cases and cocaine 10% was used in 32 cases. Localization testing with 1% hydroxyamphetamine drops was performed in 63 cases, with 29 of the patients having a preganglionic lesion and the remaining 34 patients with a postganglionic lesion. Further, 88 patients went on to have imaging to investigate for a causative lesion. The 10 patients who elected to defer imaging did so for a variety of reasons (eg, the Horner syndrome was present for many years without additional symptoms or the patient chose not to pursue imaging despite the potential for serious underlying causes). Of the 88 patients who did have imaging, 18 patients (20%) were found to have a causative lesion for their isolated Horner syndrome (**Table 1**). The most common causative lesion was a carotid artery dissection (7/88 patients). One of the imaged patients was found to have a primary malignancy, an orbital extranodal marginal zone lymphoma, and underwent focal radiation therapy. Additionally, 1 patient with known metastatic disease had a new metastatic lung lesion. Five (6%) of the 88 patients were noted to have an incidental finding on imaging, unrelated to the oculosympathetic defect, which often required additional workup (**Table 2**).

SUMMARY

In patients with isolated Horner syndrome in whom the diagnosis is not apparent from clinical history or examination, imaging of the oculosympathetic pathway is usually pursued. Our study found a causative lesion on imaging in 20% of patients with isolated Horner with unknown etiology. Almog and colleagues[6] evaluated 9 patients with isolated Horner syndrome and found a causative lesion in 1 patient, who had a thyroid carcinoma. Mollan and colleagues[7] reviewed cases of clinically isolated Horner syndrome and found causative lesions in 25 (54%) of 47 patients, with the most common identified etiology being carotid artery dissection in 11 of 47 patients. Chen and colleagues[8] found that 41% of all patients with Horner syndrome had an identifiable cause; however, this study did not require the presentation to be clinically isolated.

The most common cause of an isolated Horner syndrome in our study was a carotid artery dissection (7/88 patients). Carotid artery dissection has previously been reported as the most common identifiable cause of Horner syndrome.[7] In our study, of the 7 patients in whom a carotid artery dissection was found, all but 1 patient presented with an acute-onset painful Horner syndrome. We suggest that, unless there is associated pain at the time of presentation, emergent imaging is usually not indicated. Carotid artery dissections are the leading cause of ischemic stroke in individuals younger than 45 years, which underscores the importance of making this diagnosis. A recent review in the radiology literature suggested that MRI with MRA is the imaging modality of choice to demonstrate an intramural hematoma secondary to a carotid artery dissection.[9] Classic radiologic findings of a carotid artery dissection seen with an MRI/MRA include a hypertense T1-weighted eccentric “crescent sign” (**Fig. 2**), or narrowing of the carotid artery on MRA (**Fig. 3**), as noted in the imaging from a 44-year-old man from our study.

We found only 1 isolated Horner syndrome secondary to a primary malignancy and 1 patient with growth of a known metastatic neoplasm as a cause in our review. Other studies have found higher percentages of patients with Horner syndrome caused by a neoplasm, with 1 study reporting that approximately 17% of patients have a neoplasm as the cause.[6]

The root of this study’s question is to help determine the value of imaging in patients with isolated Horner syndrome. To our knowledge, this is the largest series evaluating the diagnostic yield of imaging for isolated Horner syndrome. Imaging identified a

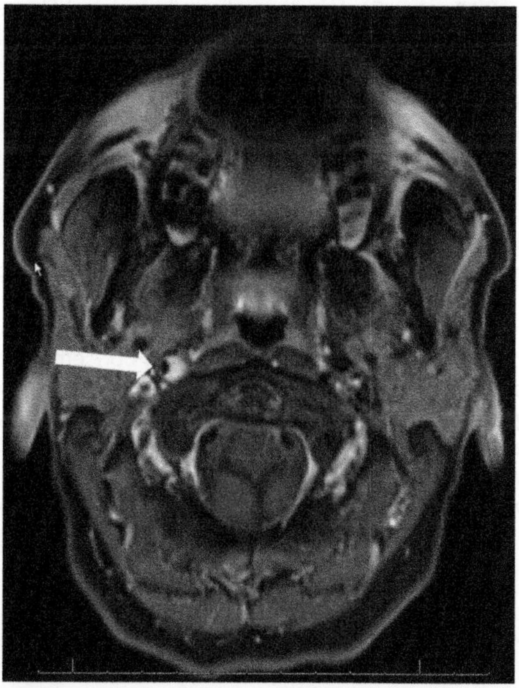

Fig. 2. Axial T1-weighted MRI with contrast image of the head and neck of a patient with isolated Horner syndrome showing the eccentric "crescent sign" (*arrow*) of the right carotid artery consistent with a carotid artery dissection.

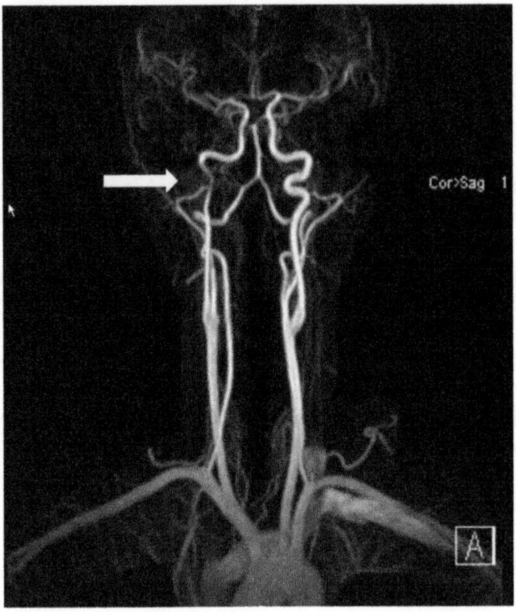

Fig. 3. MRA of the head and neck showing right carotid artery narrowing (*arrow*) consistent with a right carotid artery dissection in a patient with isolated Horner syndrome.

causative lesion in 20% of patients with a clinically isolated Horner syndrome. We found that 6% of patients had an incidental finding on imaging, unrelated to the cause of the oculosympathetic defect, which underscores the advantage of localization with pharmacologic testing to assist with radiologic interpretation.

From this study it has become more readily apparent that patients with isolated Horner benefit from radiologic investigation. Given these results for patients with isolated Horner syndrome, our institution chooses to image the entire oculosympathetic pathway and use pharmacologic localization as a mean to focus interpretation of imaging, rather than to determine the modality or extent of imaging. MRI with angiography has been the modality of choice, providing imaging of the entire oculosympathetic pathway. Patients with isolated Horner syndrome should be counseled that a significant, yet small, percentage of patients are found to have a causative lesion with imaging. Patients and clinicians are often concerned about Horner syndrome being caused by a malignancy. This study found only 1 patient with a new primary malignancy presenting as an isolated Horner syndrome. Finally, it is currently not known whether patients with isolated Horner syndrome with unrevealing imaging need to be followed over time. Presently, these patients are usually discharged and are asked to follow up only if any new signs or symptoms develop. We are currently studying the long-term outcome of these patients to determine whether there are cases in which the cause ultimately became apparent.

REFERENCES

1. Freedman KA, Brown SM. Topical apraclonidine in the diagnosis of suspected Horner syndrome. J Neuroophthalmol 2005;25(2):83–5.
2. Reede DL, Garcon E, Kardon R, et al. Horner's syndrome: clinical and radiographic evaluation. Neuroimaging Clin N Am 2008;18(2):369–385 xi.

3. Mughal M, Longmuir R. Current pharmacologic testing for Horner syndrome. Curr Neurol Neurosci Rep 2009;9(5):384–9.
4. Davagnanam I, Fraser CL, Plant GT, et al. Adult Horner's syndrome: a combined clinical, pharmacological, and imaging algorithm. Eye (Lond) 2013;27(3):291–8.
5. Digre KB, Smoker WR, Yuh WT, et al. Selective MR imaging approach for evaluation of patients with Horner's syndrome. AJNR Am J Neuroradiol 1992;13(1):223–7.
6. Almog Y, Gepstein R, Kesler A. Diagnostic value of imaging in Horner syndrome in adults. J Neuro-ophthalmol 2010;30(1):7–11.
7. Mollan S, Lee S, Senthin L, et al. Comment on 'adult Horner's syndrome: a combined clinical, pharmacological, and imaging algorithm' [letter]. Eye 2013;27:1423–4.
8. Chen Y, Morgan ML, Barros Palau AE, et al. Evaluation and neuroimaging of the Horner syndrome. Can J Ophthalmol 2015;50(2):107–11.
9. Ben Hassen W, Machet A, Rodriguez Regent C, et al. Imaging of cervical artery dissection. Diagn Interv Imaging 2014;95(12):1151–61.

Optical Coherence Tomography in Neuro-ophthalmology

Fiona Costello, MD, FRCP[a,b,*]

KEYWORDS

- Optical coherence tomography • Optic neuritis • Neuromyelitis optica
- Multiple sclerosis • Optic disc drusen • Papilledema
- Idiopathic intracranial hypertension • Pituitary tumors

KEY POINTS

- The diagnosis of many central nervous system (CNS) disorders can be facilitated through a detailed ophthalmic examination and adjunctive optical coherence tomography (OCT).
- OCT represents a surrogate marker of neuroaxonal integrity in the afferent visual pathway. Neurodegenerative components of CNS diseases can be captured with this ocular imaging technology.
- OCT should be viewed as a complement to, but not a replacement for, function visual outcomes in patients with CNS disorders.
- OCT has proved a useful tool in monitoring demyelinating disorders of the CNS, distinguishing causes of optic nerve elevation, and diagnosing pituitary tumors.

INTRODUCTION

Cardinal features of many CNS disorders can be identified through a detailed fundus examination. In the setting of raised intracranial pressure, the optic nerve may appear edematous (ie, papilledema), the severity of which has been classified according to grading scheme (eg, the Frisen scale).[1] In cases of chronic optic neuropathy secondary to compressive, ischemic, inflammatory, infiltrative, and infectious etiologies, the optic nerve often appears pale and atrophic. Retinal nerve fiber layer (RNFL) defects may manifest as a consequence of an optic nerve injury. Yet, these fundus features can be difficult to identify, even by experienced observers. In the modern era, OCT

Conflicts of Interest: None.

[a] Department of Clinical Neurosciences, University of Calgary, 1403 – 29th Street NW, Calgary, Alberta T2N 2T9, Canada; [b] Department of Surgery, University of Calgary, 1403 – 29th Street NW, Calgary, Alberta T2N 2T9, Canada
* Department of Clinical Neurosciences, University of Calgary, 1403 – 29th Street NW, Calgary, Alberta T2N 2T9, Canada.
E-mail address: Fiona.Costello@albertahealthservices.ca

Neurol Clin 35 (2017) 153–163
http://dx.doi.org/10.1016/j.ncl.2016.08.012
0733-8619/17/

complements conventional ophthalmoscopy techniques, by providing a quantitative means of capturing acute and chronic effects of optic nerve injury. The RNFL is comprised, in part, by retinal ganglion cell axons and lacks myelin. Therefore, changes in RNFL thickness have been interpreted to reflect axonal injury.[2] Within the macular region, there is a high proportion of retinal ganglion cells. Loss of macular thickness and thinning of the ganglion layer represent neuronal damage in afferent visual pathway. In recent years, OCT has emerged as a structural marker, which may facilitate understanding of mechanisms of neurodegeneration that contribute to neurologic disability in a variety of CNS diseases.

MONITORING DEMYELINATING DISORDERS OF THE CENTRAL NERVOUS SYSTEM

Acute Optic Neuritis

Optic neuritis may occur as a sporadic event or in the context of multiple sclerosis (MS). For 1 in 5 MS patients, optic neuritis represents the first clinical manifestation of their disease.[2] The Optic Neuritis Treatment Trial demonstrated that most optic neuritis patients are young (mean age: 32 years), white (85%), and women (77%) who report pain at the time of symptom onset (92%).[2–4] Vision loss tends to progress over hours to days and may range from mild (Snellen visual acuity equivalent of 20/20) to severe (no light perception) initially.[2] In patients with unilateral optic nerve involvement, a relative afferent pupil defect (RAPD) can be detected in the affected eye. In the context of bilateral optic neuritis, the RAPD localizes to the more severely affected eye but an RAPD may be absent in bilateral and symmetric disease. Patients frequently note color desaturation, referred to as dyschromatopsia, which can be disproportionate to their high-contrast visual acuity deficit.[2] In cases of retrobulbar optic neuritis, the fundus examination may appear normal, whereas patients with anterior optic neuritis (papillitis) demonstrate mild to moderate optic disc swelling.[2] Visual recovery after optic neuritis typically occurs within weeks, and the overall prognosis is favorable, with more than 90% of patients achieving a visual acuity of 20/40 after 1 year.[2–4] Despite regaining normal visual function as measured by standard ophthalmic testing, many optic neuritis patients report persistent problems with heat-induced vision loss (Uhthoff phenomenon), altered motion perception, and decreased spatial vision at low-contrast levels. There is, therefore, a need for more sensitive measures of structural injury and functional impairment in this patient population.

In the acute phase, OCT-measured peripapillary RNFL measurements are often elevated in the optic neuritis eye, presumably due to axoplasmic flow stasis.[2,5] This initial spike in RNFL thickness makes it difficult to identify the earliest signs of retrograde axonal degeneration from the retrobulbar site of optic nerve inflammation and hampers attempts to precisely tract axonal injury. In contrast, OCT-measured macular volume and ganglion layer measures are generally comparable between affected and unaffected eyes of patients at the time of symptom onset, declining for 6 to 12 months thereafter.[5] Retinal segmentation techniques have shown that in the initial months that follow optic neuritis, the percentage decrease in ganglion layer thickness correlates with increased outer nuclear layer and photoreceptor layer thicknesses, albeit these outer layer measurements subsequently decline between months 4 and 12 postevent.[6] Postacute functional outcomes (high-contrast and low-contrast letter acuity, color vision, and visual field sensitivity measures) after optic neuritis correlate with the eventual of extent of OCT-measured RNFL, ganglion layer, and macular volume loss detected 6 to 12 months after the event.[2]

Recurrent optic neuritis has been associated with worse OCT measures of neuroaxonal integrity in the afferent visual pathway. Yeh and colleagues[7] demonstrated a

9-μm (9%) decrement in RNFL thickness for each additional clinical episode of optic neuritis in a pediatric patient population with demyelinating syndromes. The presence of an OCT floor effect can make it difficult to detect appreciable changes in RNFL thickness in the setting of severe optic atrophy, or recurrent optic neuritis, because mean RNFL values do not generally decrease below a measure of approximately 30 μm regardless of the extent of optic nerve injury.[8] For this reason, I believe that it is ill advised to rely on OCT measures in isolation to track the effects of recurrent optic neuritis. Instead, I advocate that OCT measures should be interpreted in concert with other tests of afferent visual pathway structure and function, including visual evoked potentials, perimetry, color vision perception, and high/low-contrast letter acuity.

> There is a floor effect with OCT, which limits detection of progressive RNFL and ganglion layer loss in cases of recurrent optic neuritis. Therefore, OCT measures should not be interpreted in isolation.

Neuromyelitis Optica Spectrum Disorder

Neuromyelitis optica spectrum disorder (NMOSD) encompasses inflammatory syndromes of the CNS, which typically cause irreversible damage to the optic nerves and spinal cord. A disease-specific serum immunoglobulin IgG, which targets the aquaporin-4 water channel, has facilitated differentiation of NMOSD from MS, with a sensitivity of up to 80%.[9] The optic neuritis associated with NMOSD tends to be more severe than in MS. Thus, it is not surprising that OCT-measured RNFL, macular volume, and ganglion layer measurements are generally lower in NMOSD patients relative to their MS counterparts.[9] Specifically, optic neuritis has been associated with a mean RNFL loss of 20 μm in MS eyes relative to healthy controls, whereas RNFL values in NMOSD patients are reduced by 55 μm to 83 μm.[9] Compared with typical MS-related optic neuritis, OCT-measured RNFL thinning in NMOSD eyes tends to involve all of the peripapillary regions without preferential involvement of the temporal quadrant.[9] As a further distinguishing factor, MS eyes manifest reduced RNFL values, even in the absence of prior optic neuritis. In contrast, unaffected eyes of NMOSD patients have RNFL values that are comparable to healthy control subjects,[9] which suggests that damage to the afferent visual pathway is more often mediated by relapses, in lieu of subclinical neuroaxonal injury in this condition. OCT-detected microcystic macular edema is more prominent in individuals affected by NMOSD (20%–26% of patients; 40% of optic neuritis–affected eyes in AQP4-IgG–positive patients) relative to MS patients (5%).[9] The presence of microcystic macular edema is not unique to demyelinating optic neuropathies, but its preponderance in NMOSD might shed light on pathophysiologic mechanisms of CNS injury associated with the clinical syndromes included in this spectrum disorder.

> OCT features that distinguish NMOSD from MS include lower RNFL and ganglion layer values in NMOSD optic neuritis eyes; normal RNFL values in the absence of optic neuritis in NMOSD eyes; and higher prevalence of microcystic macular edema in NMOSD eyes.

Multiple Sclerosis

MS is an inflammatory disorder of the CNS, which causes progressive CNS neurodegeneration and neurologic disability over time[2]; 85% of MS patients initially present a relapsing-remitting MS (RRMS), during which time they experience episodes of neurologic dysfunction, before transitioning to a secondary progressive MS phase of the disease.[2] During this phase, secondary progressive MS patients experience neurologic decline, generally in the absence of clinically overt relapses.[2] For approximately 15% of MS patients, their clinical course is not characterized by relapses. Instead, these primary progressive MS (PPMS) patients experience insidious accumulation of neurologic disability over time.[2] One of the ongoing challenges in MS is to establish sensitive biomarkers of relapse-related and subclinical CNS injury that contribute to neurologic disability.

The role of OCT has expanded greatly in the field of MS over the past decade. The studies to date have shown that optic neuritis has a prominent impact on RNFL and ganglion layer measurements in MS eyes, which overrides the effects of MS subtype, disease duration, or immune-modulatory treatment. In a meta-analysis of time-domain OCT studies, Petzold and colleagues[10] reported that MS optic neuritis eyes had RNFL values that were approximately 20 μm lower than healthy control eyes. In eyes unaffected by prior optic neuritis, RNFL values were reduced by 7 μm in MS patients compared with disease-free controls. Efforts are currently under way to perform a similar meta-analysis of spectral-domain OCT studies. Prior time-domain OCT and more recent spectral-domain studies have shown comparable rates of annual peripapilllary RNFL thinning in MS patients.[11,12] Narayanan and colleagues[12] reported a peripapillary RNFL change measuring −1.49 μm/y in eyes unaffected by optic neuritis. Differences in annual rates of RNFL atrophy are no doubt influenced by heterogeneity in the MS patient populations studied. Highest rates of optic atrophy likely are found in RRMS patients experiencing recurrent inflammatory events, whereas inactive patients with advanced disease may manifest less change in RNFL thickness over time, in part due to the OCT floor effect. Currently, there is a 3-year prospective, multicenter, open-label, parallel group study in 350 patients with RRMS and 70 healthy volunteers.[13] The overarching aim is to evaluate changes in RNFL and neuronal layer values in RRMS patients. OCT measures will be compared with annual MRI measures of brain volume and T2 lesion load.[13] The design and randomization processes of this study will control for the variables that have hampered interpretation of rates of RNFL (and ganglion layer) thinning in many of the small observational studies to date.

Several studies have shown that OCT findings may be able to differentiate MS subtypes. Oberwahrenbrock and colleagues[14] used spectral-domain OCT to characterize inner retinal layer changes in 45 patients with clinically isolated syndromes (CISs) compared with age and gender-matched controls. Even in CIS eyes without prior optic neuritis, the ganglion layer measures were reduced, similar to optic neuritis affected eyes. In many respects, this observation is unsurprising because it is not possible to determine when MS actually begins for any patient. The main difference between many CIS patients and RRMS patients is how closely they have been evaluated for subclinical evidence of disseminated disease. Previous reports have also shown that RNFL values are abnormal in the eyes of PPMS patients, although this phenotype does not manifest clinically overt optic neuritis with same propensity as patients who have experienced RRMS.[15,16] Saidha and colleagues[17] have proposed that OCT can be used to identify a novel MS phenotype, called macular thinning predominant (MTP) MS. These patients have been described as having normal OCT measured peripapillary RNFL values, reduced macular thickness measures, and significant thinning of both the inner and outer nuclear layers, with relative sparing of ganglion cell layer thickness.[17] The so-called MTP phenotype, which represented 10% of patients in the population studied, was interpreted to demonstrate that primary retinal pathology can occur independent of optic nerve pathology in MS.[17] Yet, other investigators have challenged the MTP hypothesis on the grounds that similar OCT features can be found among RRMS, PPMS, and healthy controls.[18] Specifically, Brandt and colleagues[18] have countered that the results reported by Saidha and colleagues might have been influenced by the "a priori grouping" of patients according to their position in relation to an internal Cirrus OCT normative database, causing an artifactual clustering in the outer bounds of normally distributed data. The role of OCT in distinguishing MS subtypes needs to be further explored, by correlating inner and outer retinal layer measures with other markers of disease activity, and with a clear understanding of inherent limitations of the technology.

Robust correlations have been demonstrated between OCT measures of neuroaxonal injury and reduced scores in high-contrast letter acuity, low-contrast letter acuity, color vision, and perimetry scores in MS patients.[2,19] OCT findings have also been shown to correlate with other measures of CNS injury in this patient population. In a longitudinal study of 107 MS patients followed for a median of 46 months, ganglion layer atrophy was shown to mirror whole-brain atrophy, particularly that affecting gray matter.[20] Moreover, in a recent multicenter study involving a heterogeneous cohort of 879 MS patients, OCT-measured RNFL values of less than or equal to 87 μm were associated with a doubled risk of Expanded Disability Status Scale–determined disability worsening at any time after the first and up to the third years of follow-up. This risk increased by nearly four times after the third and up to the fifth years of follow-up.[21] There is growing evidence to suggest that OCT may be used to track manifestations of neurodegeneration that lead to permanent neurologic disability in MS. The lessons from the MS experience may expand understanding regarding the future role of OCT in the clinical surveillance patients with other neurodegenerative conditions, such as Parkinson disease and Alzheimer disease.

DISTINGUISHING CAUSES OF OPTIC NERVE ELEVATION

A common clinical challenge in neuro-ophthalmology is to distinguish papilledema from pseudopapilledema as the basis of an elevated optic disc appearance. To this end, OCT can be used with existing tools used to identify cases of buried optic disc drusen (ODD), pseuopapilledema without drusen, and raised intracranial pressure. Identifying cases of raised intracranial pressure is important, because there are potentially vision-threatening and life-threatening consequences for patients. Moreover, recognizing pseudopapilledema as the basis of an elevated optic disc appearance early in the diagnostic process helps avoid unnecessary costly and invasive tests.

Optic Disc Drusen

ODD consist of acellular intracellular and extracellular deposits that often become calcified over time.[22,23] Clinically apparent drusen of the optic nerve are estimated to occur in 0.3% of the population.[23] In approximately 75% of cases, ODD are bilateral.[23] Although drusen may occur in association with several clinical conditions, such as retinitis pigmentosa, pseudoxanthoma elasticum, and Alagille syndrome, a majority of affected individuals have no underlying ocular or systemic abnormalities.[23] ODD are often asymptomatic, yet visual field abnormalities are observed in 24% to 87% of affected adults, and progress over time.[23] Vision loss is believed to arise from mechanical stress on structures within the prelaminar scleral canal and compression of retinal ganglion cell axon, which, in turn, may lead to retrograde axonal degradation and ganglion cell death.[23] Clinically, ODD may be readily visualized at the surface of the optic disc with ophthalmoscopy, particularly when using red-free techniques. Yet, distinguishing buried ODD from papilledema sometimes is challenging (**Fig. 1**).

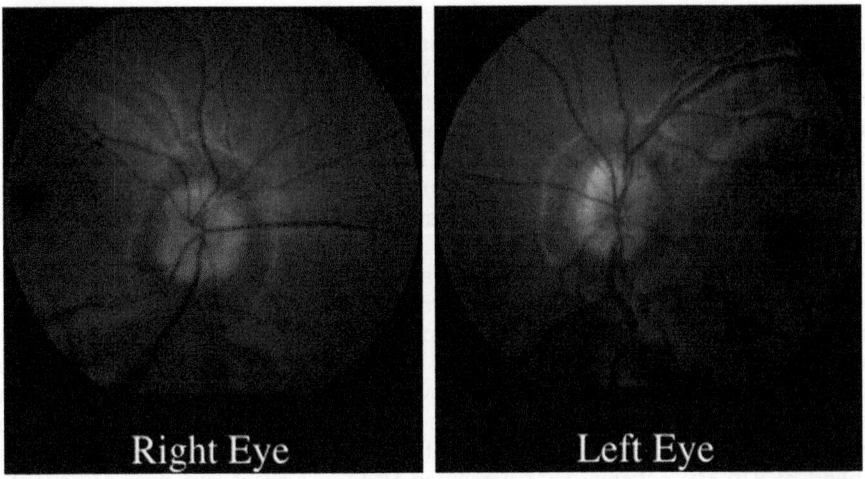

Fig. 1. Buried ODD causing optic nerve head elevation. The description Right Eye is provided directly on the fundus photo (image on the left), and the description Left Eye is directly on the optic disc photo on the right. (*Courtesy of* Dr Randy Kardon, University of Iowa, Iowa City, Iowa.)

The clinical features of buried ODD include optic disc elevation, blurred optic disc margins without obscuration of peripapillary retinal vessels, and a nodular appearance of the optic disc border.[24] In contrast, papilledema is characterized retinal nerve fiber opacification with obscuration of retinal vessels, capillary dilation over the optic disc surface, and retinal hemorrhages.[24] Key ancillary tests that can help identify cases of buried ODD include ultrasonography, fluorescein angiography, and OCT.[23,24] With B-scan ultrasonography, calcified ODD appear as highly reflective structures that can also be identified by their acoustic shadowing.[23] Because orbital ultrasound relies on calcification for detection of ODD, the sensitivity is low for noncalcified ODD.[23,24] The appearance of early or late leakage on fluorescein angiography confirms the presence of true optic disc edema, whereas buried ODD are characterized by autofluorescence, early lack of staining (75%), or early nodular staining (25%).[23,24] Moreover, buried ODD also often show late peripapillary staining—nodular (29%), circumferential (80%), or both—which is not seen in optic disc edema.[24]

OCT tends to show thinning of the RNFL and ganglion layers in cases of ODD,[25] whereas RNFL values are generally elevated in cases of papilledema. Yet simply relying on RNFL and ganglion cell layer measures as a means of distinguishing ODD from optic disc edema can be misleading, because reduced RNFL and ganglion layer measures can be observed in patients with raised intracranial pressure and coexisting optic atrophy. In attempting to define differences between RNFL in cases of buried ODD and mild papilledema, Kulkarni and colleagues[26] found no statistically significant differences between the groups. Furthermore, in this study, the ability of 5 clinicians to differentiate buried ODD from mild papilledema using the OCT images alone was poor, as was the inter-reader agreement.[26] Unfortunately, the challenge to using conventional spectral-domain OCT techniques to detect ODD is that as depth increases, the resolution of the OCT images decrease, leading to poor demarcation of deeper ODD.[23] The posterior limits of ODD are also difficult to visualize due to the hyperreflective anterior surface, which causes shadowing.[23] As an alternative, the subretinal hyporeflective space, which is located between the retinal pigment epithelium and the choriocapillaris, has been proposed as a means to detect cases of ODD.[23,27] The subretinal hyporeflective space thickness is greater in eyes with optic disc edema compared with those with drusen.[23] Other proposed methods to increase the sensitivity of distinguishing these 2 entities include enhanced-depth and swept-source OCT imaging. Enhanced-depth OCT places the coherence gate at a deeper plane than its usual position in the vitreous and moves the position of peak sensitivity from near the posterior vitreous to the inner sclera.[23] This allows visualization of structures 500 μm to 800 μm deeper than with conventional OCT testing.[23] Sato and colleagues[28] showed that enhanced OCT facilitates the assessment of shape and structure of drusen. These investigators also described a negative correlation between the diameter of ODD and RNFL thickness.[28] Similarly, swept-source OCT has been shown to significantly improve visualization of ODD, which appear as ovoid regions of low reflectivity with hyper-reflexive curvilinear borders.[23] This technique provides complete cross-sectional imaging of the ODD area and helps capture manifestations of ODD-associated RNFL thinning.[23]

> Enhanced-depth and swept-source OCT techniques can improve the diagnostic detection of buried ODD.

Papilledema Associated with Idiopathic Intracranial Hypertension

Idiopathic intracranial hypertension (IIH) is a condition of increased intracranial pressure of unknown cause, which is frequently associated with papilledema. Swelling of the optic nerve head is believed to arise from compression of the retrolaminar optic nerve, which obstructs axoplasmic flow.[29] Vision loss occurs in 86% of IIH patients, and in 10% of cases the visual deficits can be severe.[30] Causes of visual impairment in IIH patients include optic neuropathy, chorioretinal folds, hyperopic shift, hemorrhages, macular edema, and subretinal neovascularization.[31] Visual loss in IIH may be reversible if treatment is initiated in a timely fashion but can be permanent in up to 40% of patients.[31] The Idiopathic Intracranial Hypertension Treatment Trial demonstrated that acetazolamide plus weight management improved 6-month visual field outcomes in patients presenting with mild vision loss, relative to weight management plus placebo.[32] Scott and colleagues[33] have validated the role of OCT-measured RNFL thickness as a measure of papilledema severity by correlating RNFL values with Frisen-graded optic disc photos. Acutely, severe optic disc edema correlated with marked elevations in RNFL thickness and corresponding increases in macular volumes. With time and treatment, RNFL values diminish and optic disc edema abates. In chronic stages, RNFL values, macular volume and ganglion layer thickness decrease, reflecting reduced intracranial pressure with or without associated postpapilledema optic atrophy. Unfortunately, OCT is limited in the evaluation of more severe grades of papilledema, because there is an algorithm failure of the technology.[1] Sibony and colleagues[1] used OCT to show that the peripapillary retinal pigment epithelium–basement membrane, a subsurface layer that mirrors the shape of the subjacent sclera, is displaced toward the vitreous in patients with raised intracranial pressure. In a recent report, these investigators examined how lumbar puncture, cerebrospinal fluid shunting, and medical treatment of raised intracranial pressure affected the shape of the peripapillary retinal pigment epithelium–basement membrane layer.[1] They observed that patients with raised intracranial pressure had a peripapillary retinal pigment epithelium–basement membrane layer contour, which was characterized by a asymmetric shape skewed nasally toward the vitreous. In contrast, normal control subjects displayed a symmetric V shape, oriented posteriorly away from the vitreous.[1] After intracranial pressure was lowered, the peripapillary retinal pigment epithelium–basement membrane layer changed to one that appeared more V-shaped in all 3 groups, and these changes were commensurate with a decrease in the mean RNFL thickness.[1] The magnitude of the change with respect to shape, mean RNFL thickness, and displacement of the peripapillary retinal pigment epithelium–basement membrane layer was greater in patients who underwent CSF shunting, relative to patients treated medically or with lumbar puncture.[1] In patients with coexisting optic atrophy, deformations in shape did not always correlate with the severity of papilledema or RNFL thickness.[1] These findings indicated that peripapillary retinal pigment epithelium–basement membrane layer contour changes can supplement OCT-measured RNFL thickness as an indirect gauge of intracranial pressure, and may be of specific value in identifying patients with coexisting optic atrophy.[1] Sibony and colleagues[34] also used OCT to identify 3 types of folds in IIH patients with papilledema, including peripapillary wrinkles, retinal folds, and choroidal folds. Structural parameters related to the severity of papilledema were associated with peripapillary wrinkles and retinal folds, whereas anterior deformation of the peripapillary retinal pigment epithelium/basement membrane layer was associated with choroid folds and retinal folds.[34] The investigators interpreted the appearance of retinal and choroidal folds as a complex interplay between the severity of papilledema and anterior deformation of the sclera and lamina cribosa.[34]

OCT can serve as a useful tool in diagnosing cases of IIH with mild papilledema. In my experience, patients with mild grades of papilledema tend to show more variability in serial RNFL measures than expected based on test-retest parameter for OCT. Moreover, OCT measures can be useful in educating IIH patients regarding the nature of their condition and response to therapy.

DIAGNOSING PITUITARY TUMORS

Pituitary tumors are the third most common primary intracranial neoplasms with an annual incidence of 0.8 to 8 per 100,000.[35] These lesions may go undiagnosed in the absence of neuroendocrine abnormalities and/or visual dysfunction. Lesions with suprasellar extension may cause vision loss due to mass effect on the anterior visual pathway.[35] Unfortunately, loss of vision may be insidious in this context, and patients may not become aware of their deficits until late in their disease course. At this point, the potential for clinical recovery may be less promising. Visual improvement may occur after decompression (medical or surgical) of afferent visual pathway structures, albeit there are no validated predictors of recovery. Various factors that have been proposed to have an impact on postoperative visual outcomes in pituitary patients include rate of tumor growth, severity of optic chiasm compression, tumor size, preoperative OCT optical measured RNFL thickness, and duration of visual dysfunction.[35] MRI and perimetry techniques are often used to guide management of pituitary lesions. Yet, the cost, availability, and reliability of MRI in capturing clinically significant incremental tumor growth represent significant challenges. In a recent review, Ryu and colleagues[35] evaluated the utility of MRI-based structural analyses in predicting vision loss due to pituitary adenomas. In this study, MRI measures of chiasm elevation, optic nerve compression, and tumor size failed to differentiate patients with postoperative visual dysfunction from those with visual recovery after surgery. Therefore, better structural markers are needed to identify pituitary patients at risk of vision loss secondary to anterior visual pathway compression.

Several small observational studies have shown that lower preoperative OCT measures of RNFL thickness have been associated with worse visual outcomes among pituitary patients.[36,37] This finding is not surprising, because patients with preexisting structural damage to the anterior visual pathway may lack the neuroaxonal substrate required for complete visual recovery. In more recent reports, morphologic assessments of the retina and optic nerve have been performed in patients with chiasmal compression. In contrast to conventional thinking, OCT has detected structural changes in ganglion layer integrity that predate functional deficits in pituitary patients. This observation has important clinical implications because many eye care specialists perform OCT testing in patients presenting with vague visual complaints. Thus, even in the absence of classic perimetry findings of a bitemporal hemianopsia, the diagnosis of a pituitary tumor can be identified. Like glaucoma, pituitary lesions can cause slow worsening of visual function over time. Because patients with pituitary lesions may manifest optic disc cupping, occasionally these patients are wrongly diagnosed with glaucomatous optic neuropathy. Yum and colleagues[38] used spectral-domain OCT to compare ganglion layer thinning between eyes with chiasmal compression and normal or glaucomatous eyes. Their objective was to identify a specific pattern of ganglion layer involvement in eyes affected by chiasmal compression that might help localize these lesions.[38] These investigators reported a specific pattern of nasal hemiretinal ganglion layer thinning in pituitary patients without visual field defects, which should raise the index of clinical suspicion for a pituitary lesion and prompt brain imaging.[38]

SUMMARY

The evolution of OCT technology has provided a quantifiable means of capturing structural changes in retinal integrity, which can be paired with functional outcomes to follow various CNS disorders encountered in neuro-ophthalmic practice. In the future, advances in both hardware and software techniques could help advance how patients with a variety of neurologic disorders are diagnosed, monitored, and treated.

REFERENCES

1. Sibony P, Kupersmith MJ, Honkanen R, et al. Effects of lowering cerebrospinal fluid pressure on the shape of the peripapillary retina in intracranial hypertension. Invest Ophthalmol Vis Sci 2014;55:8223–31.
2. Costello F. The afferent visual pathway: designing a structural-functional paradigm of multiple sclerosis. ISRN Neurol 2013;2013:134858.
3. Beck RW, Cleary PS, Anderson MM Jr, et al. A randomized, controlled trial of corticosteroids in the treatment of acute optic neuritis. N Engl J Med 1992;326(9): 581–8.
4. Beck RW. The clinical profile of optic neuritis: experience of the optic neuritis treatment trial. Arch Ophthalmol 1991;109(12):1673–8.
5. Costello F, Pan YI, Yeh EA, et al. The temporal evolution of structural and functional measures after optic neuritis. J Neurol Neurosurg Psychiatry 2015;86(12): 1369–73.
6. Al-Louzi OA, Bhargava P, Newsome SD, et al. Outer retinal changes following acute optic neuritis. Mult Scler 2016;22(3):362–72.
7. Yeh EA, Marrie RA, Reginald YA, et al. Functional–structural correlations in the afferent visual pathway in pediatric demyelination. Neurology 2014;83:2147–215.

8. Ye C, Lam DS, Leung CK. Investigation of floor effect for OCT RNFL measurement. Invest Ophthalmol Vis Sci 2011;52(14):176.
9. Bennett JL, de Seze J, Lana-Peixoto M, et al. Neuromyelitis optica and multiple sclerosis: seeing differences through optical coherence tomography. Mult Scler 2015;21(6):678–88.
10. Petzold A, de Boer JF, Schippling S, et al. Optical coherence tomography in multiple sclerosis: a systematic review and meta-analysis. Lancet Neurol 2010;9(9): 921–32.
11. Talman LS, isker ER, Sackel DJ, et al. Longitudinal study of vision and retinal nerve fiber layer thickness in multiple sclerosis. Ann Neurol 2010;67(6):749–60.
12. Narayanan D, Cheng H, Bonem KN, et al. Tracking changes over time in retinal nerve fiber layer and ganglion cell-inner plexiform layer thickness in multiple sclerosis. Mult Scler 2014;20(10):1331–41.
13. Calabresi PA, Barkhof F, Green A, et al. RNFL as a Surrogate Outcome Marker in Patients with Multiple Sclerosis: Design of the OCTiMS study, Baseline Characteristics and OCT Test Reproducibility. April 2015; Poster Session VII Amrican Academy of Neurology: MS and CNS Inflammatory Diseases: Clinical Trials
14. Oberwahrenbrock T, Ringelstein M, Jentschke S, et al. Retinal ganglion cell and inner plexiform layer thinning in clinically isolated syndrome. Mult Scler 2013; 19(14):1887–95.
15. Pulicken M, Gordon-Lipkin E, Balcer LJ, et al. Optical coherence tomography and disease subtype in multiple sclerosis. Neurology 2007;69(22):2085–92.
16. Costello F, Hodge W, Pan YI, et al. Using retinal architecture to help characterize multiple sclerosis patients. Can J Ophthalmol 2010;45(5):520–6.
17. Saidha S, Syc SB, Ibrahim MA, et al. Primary retinal pathology in multiple sclerosis as detected by optical coherence tomography. Brain 2011;134:518–33.
18. Brandt A, Oberwahrenbrock T, Ringelstein M, et al. Primary retinal pathology in multiple sclerosis as detected by optical coherence tomography. Brain 2011; 134:1–3.
19. Sakai RE, Feller DJ, Galetta KM, et al. Vision in multiple sclerosis: the story, structure- function correlations, and models for neuroprotection. J Neuroophthalmol 2011;31:362–73.
20. Saidha S, Al-Louzi O, Ratchford JN, et al. Optical coherence tomography reflects brain atrophy in multiple sclerosis: a four-year study. Ann Neurol 2015;78:801–13.
21. Martinez-Lapiscina EH, Arnow S, Wilson JA, et al. Retinal thickness measured with optical coherence tomography and risk of disability worsening in multiple sclerosis: a cohort study. Lancet Neurol 2016;15(6):574–84.
22. Chang MY, Pineles SL. Optic disk drusen in children. Surv Ophthalmol 2016. http://dx.doi.org/10.1016/j.survophthal.2016.03.007.
23. Silverman AL, Tatham AJ, Medeiros FA, et al. Assessment of optic nerve head drusen using enhanced depth imaging and swept source optical coherence tomography. J Neuroophthalmol 2014;34(2):198–205.
24. Pineles SL, Arnold A. Fluorescein angiographic identification of optic disc drusen with and without optic disc edema. J Neuroophthalmol 2012;32(1):17–22.
25. Casado A, Rebolleda G, Guerrero L, et al. Measurement of retinal nerve fiber layer and macular ganglion cell-inner plexiform layer with spectral-domain optical coherence tomography in patients with optic nerve head drusen. Graefes Arch Clin Exp Ophthalmol 2014;252(10):1653–60.
26. Kulkarni KM, Pasol J, Rosa PR, et al. Differentiating mild papilledema and buried optic nerve head drusen using spectral domain optical coherence tomography. Ophthalmology 2014;121(4):959–63.

27. Savini G, Bellusci C, Carbonelli M, et al. Detection and quantification of retinal nerve fiber layer thickness in optic disc edema using stratus OCT. Arch Ophthalmol 2006;124:1111–7.
28. Sato T, Mrejen S, Spaide RF. Multimodal imaging of optic disc drusen. Am J Ophthalmol 2013;156:275–82.
29. Kupersmith M, Sibony P, Madel G, et al. Optical coherence tomography of the swollen optic nerve head: deformation of the peripapillary retinal pigment epithelium layer in papilledema. Invest Ophthalmol Vis Sci 2011;52:6558–64.
30. OCT Sub-Study Committee for the NORDIC Idiopathic Intracranial Hypertension Study Group, Auinger P, Durbin M, et al. Baseline OCT measurements in the idiopathic intracranial hypertension treatment trial, part I: quality control, comparisons, and variability. Invest Ophthalmol Vis Sci 2014;55:8180–8.
31. Chen JJ, Thurtell M, Longmuir RA, et al. Causes and prognosis of visual acuity loss at the time of initial presentation in idiopathic intracranial hypertension. Invest Ophthalmol Vis Sci 2015;56:3850–9.
32. The NORDIC Idiopathic Intracranial Hypertension Study Group Writing Committee, Wall M, McDermott MP, et al. Effect of acetazolamide on visual function in patients with idiopathic intracranial hypertension and mild visual loss: the idiopathic intracranial hypertension treatment trial. JAMA 2014;311(16):1641–51.
33. Scott C, Kardon R, Lee A, et al. Diagnosis and grading of papilledema in patients with raised intracranial pressure using optical coherence tomography vs clinical expert assessment using a clinical staging scale. Arch Ophthalmol 2010;128:705–11.
34. Sibony PA, Kupersmith MJ, Feldon SE, et al, OCT Substudy Group for the NORDIC Idiopathic Intracranial Hypertension Treatment Trial. Retinal and Choroidal Folds in Papilledema. Invest Ophthalmol Vis Sci 2015;56:5670–80.
35. Ryu WH, Starreveld Y, Burton J, et al. The utility of MRI in assessing patients with pituitary macroadenomas with compression of the afferent visual pathway. J Neuroophthalmol 2016. [Epub ahead of print].
36. Danesh-Meyer HV, Wong A, Papchenko T, et al. Optical coherence tomography predicts visual outcome for pituitary tumors. J Clin Neurosci 2015;22(7):1098–104.
37. Jacob M, Raverot G, Jouanneau E, et al. Predicting visual outcome after treatment of pituitary adenomas with optical coherence tomography. Am J Ophthalmol 2009;147(1):64–70.
38. Yum HR, Park SH, Park HY, et al. Macular ganglion cell analysis determined by cirrus HD optical coherence tomography or early detecting chiasmal compression. PLoS One 2016;11(4):e0153064.

Index

Note: Page numbers of article titles are in **boldface** type.

http://dx.doi.org/10.1016/S0733-8619(16)30109-8
0733-8619/17

M

N

O

V

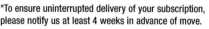

Printed and bound by CPI Group (UK) Ltd, Croydon, CR0 4YY
03/10/2024
01040388-0016